KAPLAN

Other Kaplan Books for Premedical Students

MCAT Comprehensive Review
MCAT Workbook
Medical School Admissions Adviser

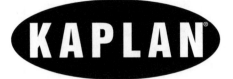

MCAT 45®

by the staff of Kaplan, Inc.

Simon & Schuster

New York · London · Singapore · Sydney · Toronto

Kaplan Publishing
Published by Simon & Schuster
1230 Avenue of the Americas
New York, NY 10020

Contributing Editors: Trent Anderson and Albert Chen
Associate Editor: Scott Johns
Project Editor: Larissa Shmailo
Cover Design: Cheung Tai
Interior Page Production: Hugh Haggerty
Production Editor: Maude Spekes
Production Manager: Michael Shevlin
Editorial Coordinator: Dea Alessandro
Executive Editor: Del Franz

Manufactured in the United States of America
Published simultaneously in Canada

March 2002

10 9 8 7 6 5 4 3 2 1

ISBN: 0-7432-2436-1

Table of Contents

This book has the latest test information and test preparation material and is up to date at the time of publication. However, sometimes changes in the test or test registration process may be instituted after publication of this book. Be sure to read carefully all the material you receive regarding this test.

If there are any important late-breaking developments—or any changes or corrections to the Kaplan test preparation materials in this book—we will post that information at kaptest.com/publishing. Check to see if there is any information posted there regarding this book.

About the Authors

Ida M. Delmendo received her B.A. in Biological Sciences and Psychology from Rutgers College, Rutgers University. A former instructor at The Johns Hopkins University Center for Talented Youth, she was also the co-creator of a calculus mentoring handbook for Rutgers University's Department of Mathematics. At Kaplan, Ida has written and edited content for Kaplan's online MCAT preparation course and served as chief contributing editor for Kaplan's *AP Biology* book. As a Kaplan curriculum developer, she has been a writer of and production manager for pre-health (MCAT, DAT, OAT, PCAT) course materials.

Tiffany Dubé, Ph.D., received her doctorate in Chemistry (Inorganic/Organometallic) from the University of Ottawa, and her B.Sc. in Chemistry and History from Laurentian University in Ontario; she was also a postdoctoral Research Fellow at Yale University's Department of Chemistry. Her numerous awards include an National Science and Engineering Research Council Industrial Research Fellowship, and a Canadian Society of Chemistry Award for Outstanding Lecture. Her publications have appeared in the *European Journal of Inorganic Chemistry* and *Organometallics*. Tiffany is the graduate curriculum developer for organic chemistry for Kaplan's MCAT team.

Rebecca E.J. Engle has been a researcher and instructor at the University of California, Berkeley College of Chemistry, as well as a researcher in private industry. Her research areas included solid phase DNA and peptide synthesis as well as organomolecular and supramolecular chemistry. A ballet dancer and former ballet instructor, Rebecca has been a curriculum developer for Kaplan's MCAT, GMAT, GRE, and LSAT courses. She received her B.A. in chemistry from the University of California, Berkeley.

Scott M. Johns has conducted research in condensed matter physics at Cornell University, and in nuclear statistical physics and supercomputing at the University of Minnesota, where he received his B.S. in physics. He was cited for his teaching skills while teaching and tutoring physics classes. He is the co-author of a paper published in *The Astrophysical Journal*. At Kaplan, Scott has been a teacher of numerous standardized test preparation courses, a trainer of Kaplan instructors, and co-writer and developer of a new comprehensive physics course. As chief premed curriculum developer, Scott leads Kaplan's MCAT team.

Karl Lee is attending the Harvard University School of Law. He is a graduate of Amherst College, where he received his B.A. and A.M. in Chemistry. At Kaplan, Karl was a member of the pre-health curriculum team. He is one of the creators of the Kaplan MCAT Course, and was co-editor of *MCAT Comprehensive Review*.

Eileen Alcock McDonnell received her B.A. in English literature from Queens College of the City University of New York, and her J.D. from Fordham University. A former fundraiser and corporate lawyer, Eileen has scored in the 99th percentile of several standardized tests, acing the verbal sections. At Kaplan, Eileen has been a contributor to the *MCAT Comprehensive Review* as well as to MCAT course materials, including the creation of new online workshops and practice tests for student use.

Nathan J. Stokes is attending the University of Michigan Medical School after receiving top scores on the MCAT. He is a graduate of Amherst College, where he received his B.A. in Physics and Chemistry. As a Kaplan curriculum developer, he designed, wrote, and edited books, tests, and course material for teaching MCAT General Chemistry content and test strategies. A former Kaplan MCAT teacher, Nathan specialized in teaching Physical Sciences. Nathan also served as a teaching assistant for Amherst College's Department of Physics, and as a researcher at the University of Michigan Department of Physics.

The Perfect Score

Ah, perfection . . .

We humans are a demanding bunch. We don't bound out of bed in the morning aspiring to mediocrity, but rather striving for perfection. The perfect mate. The perfect job. The perfect shoes to go with the perfect outfit. We head to the beach on a perfect summer day to find the perfect spot to get the perfect tan.

Webster's defines perfection as "the quality or state of being complete and correct in every way, conforming to a standard or ideal with no omissions, errors, flaws or extraneous elements."

The MCAT test makers define perfection as a score of 45.

If MCAT perfection is what you're after, then you've come to the right place. We at Kaplan have been training test takers to ace the MCAT for over 40 years. We understand your desire for the highest possible score. For those of you shooting for the moon, we salute your quest for perfection. The perfect MCAT score. The perfect medical school. The perfect career. Do we have the perfect book for you? You bet we do. You're holding it in your hands.

WHO SHOULD USE THIS BOOK

We should warn you up front: This book is not for the faint at heart. It is comprised exclusively of examples of the toughest material you're likely to see on the MCAT. No easy stuff, no run-of-the-mill strategies—just killer passages and questions, complete with Kaplan's proven techniques to help you transcend "above average" and enter the rarified arena of the MCAT elite. If you're entertaining the notion of pulling off the perfect 45, then you're going to have to face down the most brutal material the MCAT test makers have to offer. We've compiled 35 of the toughest passages and over 200 questions to help you do just that, with complete explanations every step of the way.

This book is unique in that we presume you already have a strong knowledge base in the premed curriculum; we're assuming you have excelled in your studies. Content review is not a major component of this book. Instead, this book focuses on strategies for success on the exam and practice passages, questions, and writing prompts.

Even if a perfect score is not your immediate goal, diligent practice with the difficult material in this book can help develop your skills and raise your score. If you're looking for a more fundamental introduction to the MCAT, or practice with questions ranging from easy to difficult, then we recommend working through Kaplan's *MCAT Comprehensive Review*, which covers all the necessary science for the MCAT, and provides practice sets and a full-length test.

HOW TO USE THIS BOOK

Each chapter of the book provides detailed guidelines on how to make the most of the material. Jump right to the chapter that gives you the most trouble, or work through the chapters in the order presented—it's up to you. You may want to start with chapter 2, "General Test-Taking Strategies," and from there go on to chapter 3, "Approaching the Science Sections of the MCAT," where you'll learn about the three basic types of science passages and the four basic types of questions. From there, you can go on to chapters 4–7, starting with your weakest science. Recently, the MCAT has ramped up the difficulty level of the Verbal

Reasoning portion of the test; chapter 8, "Verbal Reasoning," presents the latest thinking in Kaplan's Verbal strategies. Chapter 9, "Writing Sample," shows you how to get a T to go with that 45.

Different people have different learning styles. If after spending some time with this book, you feel that a live course with more individualized instruction and extensive opportunity for practice is what you need, consider taking a Kaplan MCAT course. If you would like more information on Kaplan's MCAT prep courses including online options, please call us at 1-800-KAP-TEST. You can also contact us on the Web at kaptest.com.

No matter what you do, try not to overload; remember, this is dense, complicated material, and not representative of the range of difficulty you'll see on test day. One thing's for sure: If you can ace this stuff, the real thing will be a breeze.

Good luck, and enjoy!

Note to International Students

Gaining admission to a U.S. medical school can be especially challenging if you are not a U. S. citizen. In recent years, fewer than 1 percent of first-year med students were non–U.S. citizens. Most of these students attended college in the United States prior to applying to medical school.

If you are an international student hoping to attend medical school in the United States, Kaplan can help you explore your options. Here are some things to think about.

- If English is not your first language, most medical schools will require you to take the TOEFL (Test of English as a Foreign Language) or provide some other evidence that you are proficient in English.
- Plan to take the MCAT; most U.S. medical schools require it.
- Begin the process of applying to medical schools at least 18 months before the fall of the year you plan to start your studies. Most programs will have only September start dates.
- You will need to obtain an I-20 Certificate of Eligibility from the school you plan to attend if you intend to apply for an F-1 Student Visa to study in the United States.
- If you've already completed medical training outside the United States, get information about taking the United States Medical Licensing Exam (USMLE).

KAPLAN INTERNATIONAL PROGRAMS

If you need more help with the complex process of medical school admissions, assistance preparing for the MCAT, USMLE, NCLEX or TOEFL, or help building your English language skills, you may be interested in Kaplan's programs for international students. These programs were designed to help students and professionals from outside the United States meet their educational and career goals. At locations throughout the United States, international students are improving their academic and conversational English skills, raising their scores on standardized exams, and gaining admission to the schools of their choice. Our staff and instructors give you the individualized attention you need to succeed. Here are some brief program descriptions:

General Intensive English

This class is designed to help you improve your skills in all areas of English and to increase your fluency in spoken and written English. Classes are available for beginning to advanced students, and the average class size is 12 students.

TOEFL and Academic English

This course provides you with the skills you need to improve your TOEFL score and succeed at an American school. It includes advanced reading, writing, listening, grammar, and conversational English. Your training will include use of Kaplan's exclusive computer-based practice materials.

English Language Self-Study Program

This program allows you to improve your English at your own pace. The books, tapes, and videos provided are for students whose skills range from beginner to intermediate.

MCAT Test-Preparation Course

In addition to test preparation for the MCAT, Kaplan offers professional counseling and advice to help you better understand the American educational system—from choosing the right medical school, to writing your application, to preparing for an interview.

Medical English Communication Review Course

This program is for international doctors and medical professionals. Lessons include mastering pronunciation, building your medical vocabulary, and developing presentation and medical writing skills. Coursework also helps you develop the English skills you will need for the CSA exam, professional interviews, and interactions with patients.

Other Kaplan Programs

Since 1938, more than 3 million students have come to Kaplan to advance their studies, prepare for entry to American universities, and further their careers. In addition to the above programs, Kaplan offers courses to prepare for the SAT, ACT, GMAT, GRE, LSAT, MCAT, DAT, USMLE, NCLEX, and other standardized exams at locations throughout the United States. For more information, contact us at:

Kaplan International Programs
700 South Flower, Suite 2900
Los Angeles, CA 90017
Phone: 800-818-9128
Fax: 1-213-892-1364
Website: www.kaplaninternational.com
Email: world@kaplan.com

Kaplan is authorized under federal law to enroll nonimmigrant alien students.
Kaplan is authorized to issue Form IAP-66 needed for a J-1 Exchange Visitor visa.
Kaplan is accredited by ACCET (Accrediting Council for Continuing Education and Training).
Test names are registered trademarks of their respective owners.

section one

GENERAL MCAT STRATEGIES

CHAPTER ONE

Introduction to the MCAT

WHAT'S REALLY BEING TESTED ON THE MCAT

As understanding the test is the key to success, in this section we'll explain the test makers' underlying purpose and principles, and briefly review how they affect your preparation for and performance on the MCAT.

The MCAT is not like the knowledge-based exams taken in high school and college. Medical schools can assess your academic prowess by looking at your transcript. Nor is it like other standardized tests you may have taken, which focused on proving your general skills.

Here's the secret: The MCAT is both a science exam *and* a critical thinking exam. All of the Verbal Reasoning questions and 80% of the questions in the science sections are passage-based. The Physical Sciences and Biological Sciences questions require interpretation of science passages, not mere regurgitation of science facts.

In recent years, many medical schools have shifted their pedagogic focus away from an information-heavy curriculum to a concept-based curriculum, with emphasis placed on problem solving, holistic thinking, and cross-disciplinary study. This trend is reflected in the MCAT. Your intellectual development—how skillfully you absorb new ideas, how quickly you build connections between ideas, how creatively you solve problems—is far more important to admission committees than your ability to recite Young's modulus for every material known to man. The schools assume they can expand your knowledge base.

The emphasis is on reasoning, critical and analytical thinking, reading comprehension, data analysis, communication, and problem-solving skills. If you make the mistake of thinking of the MCAT as a test of biology, chemistry, organic chemistry, and physics, the constant mental gear-shifting will be exhausting and counterproductive. Instead, maintain your focus on the underlying target of the test: Your thinking skills.

CONTENT AND STRUCTURE

With the goals of the test makers in mind, let's quickly review the content and structure of the test. The MCAT is nearly six hours long and consists of four scored sections: Verbal Reasoning, Physical Sciences, Writing Sample, and Biological Sciences.

The sections of the test always appear in the same order:

Morning	**Afternoon**
Verbal Reasoning	Writing Sample
10-minute break	*10-minute break*
Physical Sciences	Biological Sciences
60-minute lunch break	

Verbal Reasoning

Time: 85 minutes

Format: 65 multiple-choice questions: Approximately 9–10 passages and 6–10 questions per passage

What it tests: Critical reading, argument analysis

Verbal Reasoning may look like the "reading comprehension" sections of other standardized tests, but don't be fooled—Verbal Reasoning is much more complicated than reading comprehension. The passage subjects are written by professionals in the social sciences, the humanities, and those areas of the natural sciences not tested on the science sections of the MCAT. No outside knowledge is tested. While this section may appear less challenging than the others, the scoring is tougher. When preparing for the MCAT, Verbal Reasoning should not be neglected. Medical schools want assurance that you can draw reliable conclusions from what you read, even under pressure and time constraints.

Physical Sciences

Time: 100 minutes

Format: 77 multiple-choice questions: Approximately 10–11 passages with 4–8 questions each; 15 stand-alone questions (not passage-based)

What it tests: Basic general chemistry concepts, basic physics concepts, analytical reasoning, data interpretation

Biological Sciences

Time: 100 minutes

Format: 77 multiple-choice questions: Approximately 10–11 passages with 4–8 questions each; 15 stand-alone questions (not passage based)

What it tests: Basic biology concepts, basic organic chemistry concepts, analytical reasoning, data interpretation

Physical Sciences and Biological Sciences questions test not only your conceptual understanding of the passage and your analytical reasoning skills, but also your grasp of basic science knowledge in biology, organic chemistry, general chemistry, and physics. Medical schools need assurance that you can apply basic science knowledge to solve complex science problems.

Physical Sciences consists of approximately 50% each of physics and general chemistry, while Biological Sciences consists of approximately 50–60% biology and 40–50% organic chemistry.

Writing Sample

Time: 60 minutes

Format: 2 essay questions, 30 minutes per essay

What it tests: Critical thinking, intellectual organization, written communication skills

The Writing Sample presents you with two essay topics for which you must develop two coherent essays. The Writing Sample became a section of the MCAT in 1991 at the request of medical school admissions communities, who wanted an assessment of your independent reasoning and written communication skills.

As you can see, the MCAT is also an endurance test, with almost five hours of multiple-choice testing, one hour of writing sample, an hour or two of administrative details at both ends of the test, and three breaks (including lunch). If you can't approach it with confidence and stamina, you'll quickly lose your composure. It's important that you take control of the test.

SCORING

All multiple-choice questions are worth the same amount—one raw point—and there's no penalty for guessing. That means that you should always fill in an answer for every question, whether you get to that question or not!

Your score report will contain four separate scores—one for each section of the test. On the three multiple-choice sections—Verbal Reasoning, Physical Sciences, and Biological Sciences—the number of correct answers is counted (your raw score) and converted to a score on a 1–15 scale (with 15 being the highest) for each section. For the Writing Sample, each of your two essays is read and scored independently by two readers. The four essay scores are then added and converted into an alphabetical scale ranging from J to T.

Section	Number of Questions	Time (Minutes)	Scoring Scale
Verbal Reasoning	65	85	1–15
Physical Sciences	77	100	1–15
Writing Sample	2	60	J–T
Biological Sciences	77	100	1–15

In addition to your scaled scores, your score report will contain scaled score means, standard deviations, percentages of students receiving each scaled score for each section, and percentile rankings. These values vary slightly with each administration.

These scaled scores are what are reported to medical schools as your MCAT scores. Your score report will tell you—and your potential medical schools—not only your scaled scores, but also the national mean score for each section, standard deviations, national scoring profiles for each section, and your percentile ranking. A "Void Test" option is available on the day of the test only.

What's a Good Score?

This depends on the strength of the rest of your application and on where you want to go to school. For each MCAT administration, the average scaled scores are approximately 8 for Verbal Reasoning, Physical Sciences, and Biological Sciences, and N for the Writing Sample. You need scores of at least 10s–11s to be considered by most medical schools, and if you're aiming for the top, you've got to score 12s and above.

But you don't have to be perfect to do well. For instance, on the AAMC's Practice Test II, you could get as many as four questions wrong in Verbal Reasoning, 21 in Physical Sciences, and 16 in Biological Sciences and still score in the 80th percentile. To score in the 90th percentile, you could get as many as two wrong in Verbal Reasoning, 16 in Physical Sciences, and 11 in Biological Sciences. Even students who receive perfect scaled scores usually get a handful of questions wrong.

Here's a look at recent score profiles to give you an idea of the shape of a typical score distribution.

Verbal Reasoning		
Scaled Score	Percent Achieving Score	Percentile Rank Range
13–15	1.4	98.6–99.9
12	3.0	95.6–98.5
11	9.4	86.2–95.5
10	12.8	73.4–86.1
9	17.1	56.3–73.3
8	13.6	42.7–56.2
7	13.5	29.2–42.6
6	12.9	16.3–29.1
5	6.9	09.4–16.2
4	4.2	05.2–09.3
3	3.0	02.2–05.1
2	1.9	00.3–02.1
1	0.2	00.0–00.2
Scaled Score Mean = 7.9 Standard Deviation: 2.41		

Physical Sciences		
Scaled Score	Percent Achieving Score	Percentile Rank Range
15	0.1	99.9–99.9
14	1.0	99.0–99.9
13	2.4	96.6–98.9
12	5.0	91.6–96.5
11	8.2	83.4–91.5
10	12.8	70.6–83.3
9	14.3	56.3–70.5
8	16.9	39.4–56.2
7	15.0	24.4–39.3
6	12.3	12.1–24.3
5	6.9	05.2–12.0
4	3.8	01.4–05.1
3	1.1	00.3–01.3
2	0.2	00.1–00.2
1	0.0	00.0–00.0
Scaled Score Mean = 8.2 Standard Deviation: 2.32		

Biological Sciences		
Scaled Score	Percent Achieving Score	Percentile Rank Range
15	0.1	99.9–99.9
14	1.1	99.0–99.9
13	2.1	96.9–98.9
12	4.1	92.8–96.8
11	8.7	84.1–92.7
10	18.1	66.0–84.0
9	16.7	49.3–65.9
8	18.1	31.2–49.2
7	8.5	22.7–31.1
6	10.6	12.1–22.6
5	4.9	07.2–12.0
4	3.4	03.8–07.1
3	2.5	01.3–03.7
2	1.1	00.2–01.2
1	0.1	00.0–00.1
Scaled Score Mean = 8.4 Standard Deviation: 2.39		

Writing Sample		
Scaled Score	Percent Achieving Score	Percentile Rank Range
T	0.5	99.6–99.9
S	3.0	96.6–99.5
R	8.5	88.1–96.5
Q	19.6	68.5–88.0
P	13.7	54.8–68.4
O	13.4	41.4–54.7
N	11.4	30.0–41.3
M	18.1	11.9–29.9
L	7.1	04.8–11.8
K	2.6	02.2–04.7
J	2.1	00.0–02.1
75th Percentile = Q 50th Percentile = O 25th Percentile = M		

Registration

The MCAT is administered twice a year, in April and in August. The registration packet for both administrations (which includes the test dates) becomes available every year in late January or early February.

To register for the MCAT, pick up a registration packet (which contains important information about MCAT fees, score reporting, and how to complete the registration materials) from your premed adviser. You can also write to:

MCAT Program Office
P.O. Box 4056
Iowa City, Iowa 52243

Or, you can contact the AAMC by phone at (319) 337-1357 (Monday–Friday, 8:30 A.M. to 4:30 P.M., central daylight time) or online at www.aamc.org. Start the process as early as possible; you'll need time not only to prepare and practice for the test, but also to get all your registration paperwork done.

Other AAMC Publications

Materials released by the AAMC include *Practice Test I, Practice Test II, Practice Test III, Practice Test IV, Practice Test V,* and *Practice Items.* Other helpful publications include *Medical School Admission Requirements, MCAT Student Manual,* and the *AAMC Curriculum Directory.*

You can purchase these publications at most college bookstores or order them directly from AAMC by writing:

Association of American Medical Colleges
Attn: Membership and Publication Orders
Dept. 66
Washington, D.C. 20055

. . .or by calling (202) 828-0416, faxing (202) 828-1123, or going online to www.aamc.org.

Preparing for the MCAT

As you can see, it's important to maximize your performance on every question. Just a few questions one way or the other can make a big difference in your scaled score.

We recommend that you take one year each of biology, general chemistry, organic chemistry, and physics prior to taking the MCAT, that you review the content in this book thoroughly, and supplement it as needed from your textbooks. However, knowing these basics is just the beginning of doing well on the MCAT.

Learning and applying the Kaplan methods and strategies outlined in this book will build your skills and confidence. When you're familiar with them, practice with all the materials available from the AAMC, working consistently throughout your preparation period. You can't be assured that your actual score will be predicted by your score on any practice test, but the score you'll get on a practice test is less important than the practice itself. *Practice Test III* includes supplementary material to help you analyze your strengths and weaknesses.

Getting your best score will require lots of practice and skill building. Let's get started!

CHAPTER TWO

General Test-Taking Strategies

In this chapter, you will find general strategies for reading passages and answering questions. You will also find strategies for developing and maintaining a positive attitude, plus tips on how to be prepared for test-day conditions.

It's a good idea to read this chapter closely, even if you are already scoring well on practice tests. You will find some useful nuggets of information that can help you edge your score upward.

READING PASSAGES

You don't have to do the passages in order. Do the easiest early on, leaving the intimidating or unfamiliar for last. Also, look for the passages with more questions and do those first to maximize points.

Your goal from the outset of the passage is to figure out what the author is saying and how ideas are linked. Every passage contains a main idea, and when you're done reading, you should be able to state it in your own words. Successfully answering the questions depends on your ability to quickly glean the author's point and to map out the passage in your mind. Don't be afraid to take a few brief notes as you read—nothing lengthy. As you read through MCAT passages, try to articulate the main idea to yourself. Read actively and critically. Consider what the author is trying to say and how the ideas are communicated. Pause between paragraphs to digest what you've read and put the ideas into your own words.

When you study for college exams, you usually commit lots of data and information to memory, so that you can recite them on the test. The MCAT isn't like this at all. True, you have to master a lot of conceptual material, but you don't have to memorize complicated equations such as Bernoulli's principle, or know the value of the ideal gas constant R. When reading a passage, there is no need to commit its details to memory. You will be able to look them up in the passage when you need them. It's more important to understand why the details are there than to memorize them.

Some test takers feel more anchored as they read the passage if they've scoped out the questions first. As a general rule, it won't save you time or effort to do so.

FACING THE QUESTIONS

Be sure that you understand the question before you move to the answer choices. Otherwise, you'll be vulnerable to persuasive but incorrect choices. One of the biggest mistakes that high-scorers make when they practice MCAT questions is carelessness. Practice makes permanence: Treat every practice question as if it were the real thing.

In general, if you need an important detail on an MCAT question, it will be provided by the question or the passage. If you've followed the advice this book has to offer on how to read passages, then you will not be wasting your time when, on Test Day, you go back to the passage to look up details that you need to answer questions.

If you don't know an answer, guess! Do this while you're still working on the passage, so you won't have to reread it later. There's no penalty for wrong answers on the MCAT. Only a very few people are able to answer every single question correctly. If you get to a question that tests specific knowledge you do not possess, skim the choices carefully to see if you can glean any clues or information from them. If not, guess quickly, don't look back, and move on.

Use the structure of a Roman numeral question to your advantage. Eliminate choices as soon as you find them to be inconsistent with the truth or falsehood of a statement in the stimulus. Similarly, consider only those choices that include a statement that you've already determined to be true. Remember that you don't have to consider the statements in order. Knowing about any one of them will get you off to a great start answering the question, so if you're unsure about the first statement, go on to the second or third. You will have plenty of opportunity to practice your Roman numeral strategy on the subject practice tests in Section 2 of this book.

ANSWER GRID EXPERTISE

An important part of your MCAT test expertise is knowing how to handle the answer grid. After all, you not only have to get right answers; you also have to transfer those right answers onto the answer grid in an efficient and accurate way. It sounds simple but it's extremely important: Don't make mistakes filling out your answer grid! When time is short, it's easy to get confused going back and forth between your test book and your grid. If you know the answer, but misgrid it, you won't get credit. Here are a few methods of avoiding mistakes on the answer grid.

Always Circle the Questions You Skip

Put a big circle in your test book around the number of any question you skip (you may even want to circle the whole question itself). When you go back, such questions will then be easy to locate. Also, if you accidentally skip an oval on the grid, you can easily check your grid against your book to see where you went wrong.

Always Circle the Answers You Choose

Circle the correct answers in your test booklet, but don't transfer the answer to the grid right away. Circling your answers in the test book will also make it easier to check your grid against your book.

Grid Five or More Answers at Once

Don't transfer your answers to the grid after every question. Transfer your answers after every five questions or at the end of each passage (find the method that works best for you). That way, you won't keep breaking your concentration to mark the grid. You'll save time and improve accuracy. Just make sure you're not left at the end of the section with ungridded answers!

Save Time at the End for a Final Grid Check

Make sure you have enough time at the end of every section to make a quick check of your grid, to make sure you've got an oval filled in for each question in the section. Remember that a question left blank has no chance of earning a point, but a guess does.

PACING

Remember that every question is of equal value, so don't get hung up on any one of them. Think about it—if a question is so hard that it takes you a long time to answer it, chances are you may get it wrong anyway. In that case, you'd have nothing to show for your extra time but a lower score, and less time for other questions.

Don't feel that you have to understand everything in a passage before you go on to the questions. You may not need a deep understanding to answer questions, since a lot of information may be extraneous. You should overcome your perfectionism and use your time wisely.

If you do the math, you will see that you have about nine minutes per passage. However, don't hold fast to a "nine minutes per passage" rule. On Test Day, some passages will be harder and longer, and others easier and shorter. A better strategy is to allow 27 minutes for three passages.

BASIC PRINCIPLES OF GOOD TEST MENTALITY

Knowing the test content arms you with the weapons you need to do well on the MCAT. But you must wield those weapons with the right frame of mind and in the right spirit.

Test Awareness

To do your best on the MCAT, you must always keep in mind that the test is like no other test you've taken before, both in terms of content and in terms of the scoring system. If you took a test in high school or college and got a number of the questions wrong, you wouldn't receive a perfect score. But on the MCAT, you can get a handful of questions wrong and still get a "perfect" score. The test is geared so that only the very best test takers are able to finish every section. But even these people rarely get every question right.

What does this mean for you? Well, just as you shouldn't let one bad passage ruin an entire section, you shouldn't let what you consider to be a subpar performance on one section ruin your performance on the entire test. If you allow that subpar performance to rattle you, it can have a cumulative negative effect, setting in motion a downward spiral. It's that kind of thing that could potentially do serious damage to your score. Losing a few extra points won't do you in, but losing your cool will.

Remember, if you feel you've done poorly on a section, don't sweat it. Chances are it's just a difficult section, and that factor will already be figured into the scoring curve. The point is, remain calm and collected. Simply do your best on each section, and once a section is over, forget about it and move on.

Confidence

Confidence feeds on itself, and unfortunately, so does the opposite of confidence—self-doubt. Confidence in your ability leads to quick, sure answers and a sense of well-being that translates into more points. If you lack confidence, you end up reading the sentences and answer choices two, three, or four times, until you confuse yourself and get off track. This leads to timing difficulties, which only perpetuate the downward spiral, causing anxiety and a tendency to rush in order to finish sections.

If you subscribe to the MCAT mindset we've described, however, you'll gear all of your practice toward the major goal of taking control of the test. When you've achieved that goal—armed with the principles, techniques, strategies, and approaches set forth in this book—you'll be ready to face the MCAT with supreme confidence. And that's the one sure way to score your best on Test Day.

The Right Attitude

It may sound a little dubious, but take our word for it: Attitude adjustment is a proven test-taking technique. Here are a few steps you can take to make sure you develop the right MCAT attitude:

- Look at the MCAT as a challenge, but try not to obsess over it; you certainly don't want to psyche yourself out of the game.
- Remember that, yes, the MCAT is obviously important, but, contrary to what some premeds think, this one test will not single-handedly determine the outcome of your life.
- Try to have fun with the test. Learning how to match your wits against the test makers can be a very satisfying experience, and the reading and thinking skills you'll acquire will benefit you in medical school as well as in your future medical career.
- Remember that you're more prepared than most people. You've trained with Kaplan. You have the tools you need, plus the know-how to use those tools.

THE DAY BEFORE TEST DAY

This is not the time to be working on a new full-length practice test—relax! Instead of studying, do something fun but low-key. Make sure that you know how to get to the test center; rehearse the drive, if necessary. Have a quiet, relaxing evening, and go to bed early.

TEST DAY: THE COMFORT ZONE

The MCAT is a day-long exam. Get a good night's sleep the evening before the exam. Wake up early, so that you aren't rushed. Prepare your admission ticket, appropriate identification, no. 2 pencils, black pens, and erasers. Dress in layers, since it may be warmer or cooler in the testing room than you would prefer. While eating breakfast on the morning of the MCAT, jump-start your brain by reading something unrelated to the test. Bring a healthy snack to the test, since you might be hungry during the midmorning break. You won't be able to eat or drink during the test. Be sure to arrive at the exam no later than 8:00 A.M.

During your lunch break, wake up your writing skills by getting a little bit of practice, as Writing Sample will be the next section of the test. Finally, don't let others intimidate you or discourage you by their words or actions. People will be chattering nervously, talking about how easy something was, or how they finished early. Remember that it's correct answers that count, not speed, and that different test forms are used, so your neighbor may have different questions than you do.

With these strategies in mind, let's now turn to the test itself for specific approaches for handling each section.

section two

PHYSICAL SCIENCES AND BIOLOGICAL SCIENCES

CHAPTER THREE

Approaching the Science Sections of the MCAT

In the last section, we took a look at the MCAT, gave some advice for coping with stress, and learned some general test-taking strategies. In chapters 6–9 of this section, we will focus on the science portions of the MCAT, providing specific advice for reading the passages and handling the questions associated with each of the four sciences. Each chapter contains seven practice passages that will allow you to put this advice into practice. Concluding each chapter is a list of specific concepts and skills you should have mastered before Test Day.

In this chapter, we offer some general advice for tackling science passages and questions. But first, let's review the structure of the two science sections on the MCAT: Physical Sciences and Biological Sciences.

THE SCIENCE SECTIONS

The Physical Sciences and the Biological Sciences sections each last 100 minutes. Each has 77 questions: 15 discrete questions, which stand alone from passages, and 62 passage-based questions. Each section has 10–11 (usually 11) passages. The Physical Sciences section usually splits evenly, with 38–39 Physics questions and 38–39 General Chemistry questions. However, the split between Biology questions and Organic Chemistry questions in the Biological Sciences section isn't always the same. Typically, the questions split 60–40 in favor of Biology; however there is a trend in recent MCATs towards a more even distribution.

In the last section, we gave some general advice on how to handle MCAT passages. On the science portions of the test, it is true that having a core knowledge in the basic concepts in the four sciences on the MCAT is very important to scoring well on Test Day. However, shrewd, sophisticated premedical students will want the extra edge needed to maximize their MCAT score. It is the purpose of the remainder of this book to provide you with that edge.

What we're talking about is test-taking strategy. Not just "eat a good breakfast" and "don't burn out before Test Day" (both of which happen to be good pieces of advice), but specific pearls of wisdom broken down by science (with corresponding advice for Verbal Reasoning and the Writing

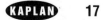

Sample to follow in Section Three.) Many people see the MCAT as purely a content-based test: know your stuff and a good score should follow. Those people are surprised to learn that, in general, they should read a Physics passage much differently than an Organic Chemistry passage.

Test-taking strategy on the science portions of the MCAT can be broken down into two major areas: Absorbing the passages, and handling the questions. Before diving into science-specific advice in subsequent chapters, let's build a framework around these two ideas.

ABSORBING THE MCAT SCIENCE PASSAGE

Passage Types

One of the first things you'll want to do when absorbing a science passage is to identify what type of passage you're reading. MCAT science passages fall into three broad categories:

> *Information*
>
> *Experiment*
>
> *Persuasive Argument*

Information passages resemble a textbook. They often include diagrams, but are largely paragraphs of dry description. Information passages describe natural or man-made phenomena.

Here's an example of an Organic Chemistry information passage:

> Aspirin, also known as acetylsalicylic acid, is one of the most useful and economical drugs available. It belongs to a class of drugs known as nonsteroidal anti-inflammatory drugs, and can be used to treat pain and alleviate inflammation and fever. The mechanism of aspirin's action is not fully understood, although recent research suggests that it functions by inhibiting cyclooxygenase 2, an enzyme that creates prostaglandin precursors. Prostaglandins contribute to the body's perception of pain and its inflammatory response. Prostaglandins also aid in the formation of blood clots, so aspirin thins the blood and may consequently help prevent heart disease.
>
> Aspirin can be synthesized from salicylic acid via the reaction shown in Figure 1.

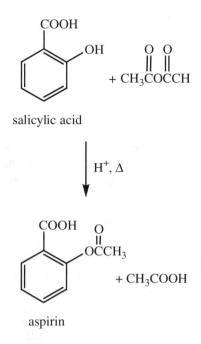

salicylic acid

aspirin

Both salicylic acid and aspirin are aromatic carboxylic acids. Carboxylic acids are generally weak acids, although they are among the strongest organic acids, with pK_a's usually in the range of 3 to 5, much lower than those of corresponding alcohols. The pK_a's of some compounds are given in Table 1.

Table 1 pK_a's of Compounds

Compound	pK_a
Acetic acid	4.76
Fluoroacetic acid	2.66
Difluoroacetic acid	1.24
Trifluoroacetic acid	0.23
2,2-Dimethylpropanoic acid	5.05
Benzoic acid	4.18
p-Nitrobenzoic acid	3.43
2,4,6-Trinitrobenzoic acid	0.65
p-Methoxybenzoic acid	4.47
Phenol	9.95
Ethanol	15.9
Methanol	15.1
Water	14

Experiment passages describe one (or more) experiments, and have clear goals. Something is varied, something else is measured, and conclusions can be formed. Sometimes an experiment passage focuses on a table or a graph giving the results of the experiment, and sometimes the passage focuses on the experimental apparatus.

This is an example of a Physics experiment passage:

The mass spectrometer is a device that utilizes electric and magnetic fields to determine the masses of the elements or compounds that exist within a certain sample. The operation of the mass spectrometer relies on the fact that the path of a moving charge is affected by the presence of electric and magnetic fields.

To analyze a sample, it must first be ionized. This may be accomplished by bombarding it with a stream of electrons. The ionized particles are then accelerated through a potential difference of several thousand volts that is set up between two slits S_1 and S_2 (see figure below). For the mass spectrometer to give useful results, all the particles entering the chamber below S_3 must be traveling at the same velocity. This is assured by passing the particles through a *velocity selector*, a region of a crossed magnetic field, B, and an electric field, E, located between S_2 and S_3. This electric field is produced by two charged parallel plates, P_1 and P_2. Only particles that are traveling at a velocity such that the force due to the electric field (qE) and that due to the magnetic field (qvB) cancel one another will remain undeflected and pass through the slit in S_3.

The stream of charged particles then pass though another magnetic field, B', but this time, there is no electric field. The second magnetic field is perpendicular to the page, and deflects the particles in a circular path, towards the detector. Based on the radius of curvature of the path of the particle, its mass can be determined from the formula:

$$\frac{q}{m} = \frac{E}{rBB'}$$

where q is the charge of the particle, m is the mass of the particle, E is the electric field, and r is the radius of the circular path of the particle. In the mass spectrometer below, $E = 8 \times 10^4$ V/m, 0.4 T, and $B' = 0.5$ T. The fundamental unit of charge is 1.6×10^{-19} C.

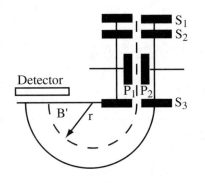

Figure 1   Mass Spectrometer

Persuasive argument passages present contrasting viewpoints on a subject. The typical format is for the passage to introduce a phenomenon, and then present the differing viewpoints or hypotheses. Answering many of the accompanying questions correctly will then rely on your understanding the similarities of and the differences between the hypotheses.

The following is an example of a Biology persuasive argument passage:

> *Alzheimer's disease* is a neurological condition that results in degeneration of the brain. Two forms of the disease exist: a hereditary form, which is characterized by early onset of symptoms, usually when the patients are in their forties, and a late-developing form of the disease, called senile dementia, which may not be of genetic origin. Two current hypotheses describing possible mechanisms of hereditary Alzheimer's disease are outlined below.
>
> *Hypothesis A*
> Alzheimer's disease is a result of a mutation in the gene encoding amyloid precursor protein (APP). APP usually gives rise to a smaller protein known as beta amyloid, which is a major component of the abnormal plaques that are a feature of Alzheimer's pathology. The presence of these plaques is the cause of the neuronal deterioration associated with the disease.
>
> The mutation results in the insertion of an isoleucine residue in place of a valine residue. The mutation interferes with normal APP function, causing membrane degeneration and enhancing beta amyloid release. The increase in beta amyloid release promotes the formation of the Alzheimer's-causing plaques.
>
> *Hypothesis B*
> Alzheimer's disease is a result of a mutation in the gene encoding a protein called *acetylcholinesterase*, the enzyme responsible for the breakdown of the neurotransmitter acetylcholine. A comparison of the abnormal acetylcholinesterase to the normal acetylcholinesterase reveals that the mutant enzyme is 30 amino acids shorter. The mutation inactivates acetylcholinesterase, resulting in a build-up of acetylcholine in the neurons. A high level of acetylcholine blocks impulse transmission from one neuron to another, resulting in a loss of cholinergic nerve terminals in the cerebral cortex; thus, Alzheimer's disease is promoted. The consequence of cholinergic nerve degradation is a build-up of beta amyloid-containing plaques.

Reading the Passage

One of the traps that many test takers fall into is spending too much time reading the passages. They waste effort trying to retain every fact and detail introduced, and to understand every aspect of the phenomenon or experiment described. This is especially true of students who have performed very well in school, who expect to master everything. However, this type of reading will *not* pay off on an MCAT science passage.

First, keep in mind that the same passage may appear on different test forms *with slightly different sets of questions*. So, something that baffles you may not even be touched upon by the questions. There is certainly no point in wasting time trying to figure out something that ultimately does not win you any points on the test. Second, the data and information from the passage are always there if you need them. For example, the mass of the block sliding down an inclined plane, the melting point of an unknown compound isolated in a reaction, or the value of the gas constant R can be retrieved from the passage *when you need it to answer a question*.

Mapping the Passage

The key to efficient, critical reading of an MCAT science passage lies in creating a *passage map*. The idea of mapping a passage lies *in reading for structure*. Instead of trying to memorize everything, take a broad look at what is happening in the passage. Come out of each paragraph with a grasp on what is going on. Identify the role of each "structural component" of the passage by asking yourself: "What is this diagram/table/equation doing here?" At the beginning of your MCAT preparation, you should write down the main idea of each paragraph explicitly next to the text. You can wean yourself off written notes as you become more and more comfortable with the technique. Furthermore, you should annotate the passage by circling key definitions, etc.

The technique of mapping a passage and annotating key elements will be illustrated for each of the four science areas and for each passage type in subsequent chapters.

Identifying the Topic

In addition to mapping the passage, you should also identify the topic of the passage. However, determining the topic involves more than just coming up with a scientific term corresponding to the main subject of the passage. To identify the topic, you should answer the question, "What is the author trying to accomplish in this passage?" Being able to formulate an answer to this question means that you have read the passage critically. The answer to this question is what we mean by the topic of the passage.

The topic of a passage is related to the passage type. For an information passage, for example, the topic usually takes the following form:

> *The passage describes/discusses …*

The topic of an experiment passage can usually be phrased as:

> *The passage is about an experiment, the purpose of which is to …*

The topic of a persuasive argument passage usually has the form:

> *The passage presents (some number of) hypotheses about …*

Handling the Questions

Once we have made our passage map, we'll begin handling the questions. The first thing to do as we encounter a question is to classify it. This step is crucial, as it will help us answer the question in the quickest, most efficient manner. Each question will fall into one of the following four categories:

1. Discrete questions
2. Questions that require an understanding of the passage
3. Questions for which we need only data from the passage
4. Questions that can stand alone from the passage

Let's discuss these question types and look at an example of each.

1. Discrete questions are those that do not follow any passage and are always preceded by a header such as "Questions 121 through 127 are NOT based on a descriptive passage." Since they do not accompany a passage, all the information needed to answer these questions will be found in the question stem, the answer choices and your outside knowledge. For example, to answer the following question, you need only your outside knowledge of periodic trends:

> Which of the following properties generally decreases as one goes from left to right across the periodic table?
>
> A. Number of neutrons
>
> B. Electronegativity
>
> C. Atomic weight
>
> D. Atomic radius

The final three question types will always follow a passage:

2. Questions that require an understanding of the passage cannot be answered without having read the passage. These questions usually follow experiment or persuasive argument passages, though they may follow information passages. A question may ask us to evaluate experiments or hypotheses presented in the passage and will require us to have a conceptual understanding of topics discussed in the passage. For example, it would be virtually impossible to answer the following question correctly if we had not closely read the passage about Alzheimer's disease:

> In which of the following ways does Hypothesis A differ from Hypothesis B?
>
> A. Hypothesis A describes the mechanism of hereditary Alzheimer's; Hypothesis B describes the mechanism of senile dementia.
>
> B. Hypothesis A argues for the formation of beta amyloid-containing plaques; Hypothesis B argues against the formation of beta amyloid-containing plaques.
>
> C. Hypothesis A assumes beta amyloid-containing plaques are the cause of Alzheimer's; Hypothesis B assumes beta amyloid-containing plaques are the result of Alzheimer's.
>
> D. Hypothesis A claims that neuronal cells deteriorate in Alzheimer's; Hypothesis B claims that neuronal cells are only rendered dysfunctional.

We may have some outside knowledge of Alzheimer's disease, but reading the passage is still the best way to answer this question, since our outside knowledge may or may not be applicable to the specific hypotheses presented in this passage. For questions that require knowledge of the passage, we must adhere to the logic of the passage, even if it contradicts our outside knowledge.

3. Questions for which we need only data from the passage are similar to understanding questions in that the passage provides necessary information, but in this case, we need only refer to the passage for a piece of data. We are not required to have read the surrounding prose in order to answer these questions correctly. We will usually be referring to a table or an equation. One example of this type of "data question" could follow the physics passage we read about the mass spectrometer:

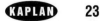

What is the force on a singly charged ion due to the electric field between plates P_1 and P_2?

A. 6.4×10^{-20} N

B. 8.0×10^{-20} N

C. 8.0×10^{-15} N

D. 1.3×10^{-14} N

In order to answer this question, we need to refer to the data in the passage, but we don't need to have read or understood the prose in the passage. Once we have found the piece of data we need, we can just plug it in to whatever equations and formulas we are using to get the correct answer.

4. Questions that can stand alone from the passage ("pseudodiscretes") are those that follow a passage but are in all other ways discrete questions. They require absolutely no knowledge of information from the passage, and are only related to the passage by their subject. The following question, for example, could follow the passage we read earlier about aspirin:

Which of the following best accounts for the higher acidity of phenol compared to ethanol?

A. Phenol is hydrophobic.

B. Phenol has a higher molecular weight.

C. The benzene ring of phenol stabilizes negative charge.

D. The oxygen atom in phenol is sp^2-hybridized.

Even though this question follows the aspirin passage, it is basically a discrete question about the acidity of organic compounds. No knowledge of the passage is necessary to answer it correctly.

Answering the Questions

When answering the questions, go through the following steps:

- Understand what you are being asked.
- Figure out where to go to get any information that you need.
- Integrating your science knowledge with any necessary passage research, determine the correct answer.

Understand what you are being asked.

The first thing to do is read the entire question, including the answer choices. Reading the answer choices can help you focus your thoughts if the question stem by itself doesn't look particularly manageable. Using your reading comprehension skills, simplify the question to its bare essentials. Translate the question into your own words if necessary. Use the answer choices to help you. Does the question ask for a numerical answer (e.g., "What is the tension in the rope?"), a distinct piece of information (e.g., "What type of reaction is illustrated in the figure below?"), or a sentence (e.g., "Why did the scientist add liver extract to the sample in Experiment 2?")?

Let's look at one of the sample questions presented earlier.

> What is the force on a singly charged ion due to the electric field between plates P_1 and P_2?
>
> A. 6.4×10^{-20} N
> B. 8.0×10^{-20} N
> C. 8.0×10^{-15} N
> D. 1.3×10^{-14} N

Simplify/translate the question: what is it asking? Here you are asked to calculate the force due to an electric field on a particle.

Figure out where to go to get any information that you need.

Do you have enough information to answer the question? Do you need information from the passage? If so, where in the passage can you find it? From your map of the passage, you should be able to quickly locate any information that you may need.

> What is the force on a singly charged ion due to the electric field between plates P_1 and P_2?
>
> A. 6.4×10^{-20} N
> B. 8.0×10^{-20} N
> C. 8.0×10^{-15} N
> D. 1.3×10^{-14} N

To calculate the force due to an electric field on a particle, you need to know the formula for the force on an electric charge in an electric field (outside knowledge). You also need to know the electric field strength and the charge on a singly charged ion—both provided by the passage. From your passage map, you should know where to get this information.

Integrating your science knowledge with any necessary passage research, determine the correct answer.

This is the step where you bring together all the previous steps together with your science knowledge to determine the correct answer. Prior to arriving at this step, you need to understand what you are being asked and gather any information you may need from the passage. Once these tasks are accomplished, use your reasoning and/or calculation skills together with your science knowledge to arrive at the answer.

Try to formulate your own explanation before going through the answer choices.

What is the force on a singly charged ion due to the electric field between plates P_1 and P_2?

A. 6.4×10^{-20} N

B. 8.0×10^{-20} N

C. 8.0×10^{-15} N

D. 1.3×10^{-14} N

$E = \dfrac{F}{q}$ $F = qE$

From your outside knowledge of physics, recall that the formula needed in this case is $F = qE$, where q is the charge on a singly charged ion and E is the electric field strength. From the passage, q is 1.6×10^{-19} C and the electric field strength is $E = 8 \times 10^4$ V/m. Carrying through the calculation, we get 1.28×10^{-14} N, which is closest to choice **D**.

 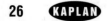

CHAPTER FOUR

Physics

The one thing that you want to keep in mind as you tackle the Physics passages is that the MCAT is only asking you to apply a basic set of physics principles. The test certainly isn't asking you to push the boundaries of known science. As a result, your success on the Physics questions on the MCAT will depend in large part on your *mastery* of the concepts of physics. At the end of this chapter is a list of the physics skills and concepts you should have in your arsenal by Test Day.

But while mastery of physics is an important ingredient to MCAT success, it isn't the only ingredient. You will want to be familiar with the test, with how the physics is tested. The better prepared you are for what you are going to see, the more confident you will feel on Test Day. The purposes of this chapter are to show you how the MCAT sets up Physics passages, to show you what kinds of Physics questions to expect, and to describe an efficient, time-saving method for tackling both Physics passages and Physics questions on Test Day.

READING THE PASSAGE

One of the worst things you can do as a test taker is to approach a Physics passage with an attitude such as, "I'm going to read this entire passage, memorizing all the details and data points as I go along, so that I won't need to waste time referring to the passage while I answer the questions." You don't want to spend most of your time reading the passage; you'd be much better off spending the bulk of your time thinking about the questions. You won't get any points for knowing the passage. Remember that the MCAT is asking you to apply what you know to the topic at hand. For some questions, the topic of the passage won't even be important; you'll simply need to apply what you know.

Passage Types

One of the first things you'll want to do is to identify what type of passage you're reading. Physics *information* passages describe natural (fission of uranium nuclei, supernovae) or man-made (sledding down a hill, standing waves in a laser cavity) physical phenomena. Look out for definitions of new terms. Roughly half of Physics passages on the MCAT are information passages.

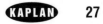

The other half of Physics passages are *experiment* passages. Physics passages that carry out an experiment (or multiple experiments) have clear goals. Something is varied, something else is measured, and conclusions can be formed. Sometimes these passages focus on a table or a graph giving the results of the experiment, and sometimes the passage focuses on the experimental apparatus. When multiple experiments are performed, be aware of the similarities and differences between the experiments: If making a small change to an experiment creates a radically different result, you can bet that there will be a question whose solution will require you to understand what the causes are. You saw an example of a Physics experiment passage in the last chapter.

Physics *persuasive information* passages are very rare. When physicists disagree as to the nature of a phenomenon, the argument pertains to those laws of physics that are too advanced to be tested on the MCAT. You won't see two scientists arguing about whether or not Newton's Second Law applies to a scenario.

As you prepare for the MCAT, remember that your skill at absorbing what needs absorbing, and skimming over what can be skimmed over will directly translate into time saved and more points on Test Day. With that in mind, here are two things to always do when reading a Physics passage.

Map the Passage

As previously mentioned, you shouldn't read a passage trying to memorize everything. Instead, you should employ your critical reading skills. You want to come out of each paragraph knowing its gist. One way of thinking about this is to ask yourself, after every paragraph, "What is this paragraph doing? Why is it here?"

The degree of detail you need to absorb depends on the type of passage. Since it isn't always immediately obvious what type of passage you are reading, you should quickly attempt to determine the passage type as you start reading any passage. Since there are only two major types of Physics passage, with practice you should be able to quickly figure this out. Once you know the passage type, then you'll know how to read it, as we discuss presently.

In an information passage, all you need to know from each paragraph is a general idea of what's being discussed. Since each paragraph will be a dry recounting of information, simply learning what's being talked about will be sufficient.

In an experiment passage, you will want to pay close attention to the manner in which an experiment is carried out. This is in contrast to Organic Chemistry passages, where the laboratory details of complicated chemical syntheses are unimportant. After Physics experiment passages, there will be at least one question asked which depends on your detailed understanding of how the experiment is done. What is the goal of the experiment(s)? What is being tested? Which variables are held constant, and which variables are changing? It's not necessary for you to memorize data points, or data from tables or graphs. If you happen to notice any general trends, so much the better, but don't worry about it too much at this stage. You can come back for data points later, if a question calls for it.

In a persuasive argument passage, you'll want to pay close attention to two things: the phenomenon being discussed, and the contrasting arguments cited. Questions can focus on the subtle difference between hypotheses, or can be tightly focused on one hypothesis.

Another common way for the MCAT to present information in a Physics passage (of any type) is to devote a paragraph to defining something. Many times a new equation will be introduced. In circumstances like this, the test makers are announcing their intention to make you use this information in a question. What you don't want to do is circle the equation or term; instead, circle the phrase or sentence that describes what the equation or term *means* or *does*. For example, imagine this paragraph thrown in at the end of a passage:

The magnetic force per unit length on two current carrying wires is $\frac{\mu_0 I_1 I_2}{2\pi a}$, where a is the distance between the two wires, I_1 and I_2 are the currents in each wire, and $\mu_0 = 4\pi \times 10^{-7} \frac{N}{A^2}$ is the permeability of free space.

Now, when a question asks about the magnetic force between two wires, you will know exactly where to go! The underlined information that describes the equation is what you want to make note of, instead of committing the equation to memory.

Whether or not you take written notes as you read a passage depends on your comfort level. We recommend that you annotate you passages as you begin to practice reading them, and then wean yourself off of annotating as you feel comfortable keeping all the needed information in your head. Maybe you'll discover that annotating passages is a great help to you, and you'll decide to keep doing it right up through Test Day. Either way, it's up to you. As you annotate, be sure to summarize each paragraph, underlining the meanings of new terms or equations, as discussed above. Your notes for each paragraph usually don't need to be much more than a few words to a sentence.

Identify the Topic

Once you have finished reading a passage, you'll want to be able to answer the question, "What is the author trying to accomplish in this passage?" Being able to answer this question means that you have read the passage critically—and critical reading is the most important skill for reading MCAT passages. The answer to this question provides the *topic* of the passage.

While determining the topic, you will also want to identify what Physics *concepts* are involved in the passage. It stands to reason that if the MCAT chooses a passage in which a mass oscillates on the end of a spring, there will be at least a few questions covering periodic motion. It is worth your time to take a few seconds to review in your mind what science the questions might cover. This exercise will help you focus and understand what you just read, and will prepare you for at least a good fraction of the questions to follow.

This is not good advice to follow for the other sciences. Physics passages are unique, because you can, by connecting what was discussed to the concepts you learned in class, predict the nature of some of the questions that follow.

This step will be particularly helpful for experiment passages; the physics concepts involved will dictate the results of the experiment. For example, say the goal of the experiment in a passage is to measure the current in a simple circuit as different resistors are inserted. The concept behind this is Ohm's Law, $V = IR$. You'd expect the voltage, different resistances, and the circuits to follow Ohm's Law every time. Perhaps there will be a question about power ($P = IV$); or maybe different groups of resistors will be hooked up in series or parallel.

Don't take more than a few seconds to think about concepts, however. The concepts you're going to be tested on are already in front of you, in the questions themselves. The odds are good that the MCAT is going to ask you at least one question about something you couldn't have anticipated—so don't spend more than a few seconds trying!

Over the next two pages are examples of how to read the two major passages types in Physics, the information passage and the experiment passage. Starting with the following information passage, read the passage, and think carefully about the passage map as you read the comments that follow them.

> Progress in the field of cellular and subcellular systems is made possible by compound microscopes. These multiple-lens instruments magnify objects that would otherwise be undetectable to the human eye. A compound microscope is composed of two converging lenses, the objective and the eyepiece. The objective forms a real image of the object. This image is then magnified by the eyepiece, which functions as a simple magnifier. The image formed by a simple magnifier is virtual, erect, and farther from the magnifier than the object. The overall magnification of the microscope is the product of the magnifications of the eyepiece and the objective.

Your annotations may read: Information passage—lenses in microscopes. This paragraph describes the two lenses in a microscope.

> The specimen to be magnified by the microscope is set on a support known as the stage. The stage is located just beyond the focal length of the objective lens. Light from a lamp and mirror arrangement illuminates the specimen from below. The light that passes through the specimen enters the objective lens, and the image produced is an enlarged, inverted image of the specimen. The image produced by the objective serves as the object for the next lens, the eyepiece. This second lens further enlarges the image, but does not invert it.

Second paragraph: Describes how a microscope works—not important to learn the details now.

> A specific example of the use of microscopes occurs in cellular biology, where scientists often use fluorescently labeled proteins to highlight different regions of a cell. In a special microscope equipped with a fluorescent lamp (which radiates light in the ultraviolet region of the spectrum), the areas of interest can be identified by observing the brightly colored areas where the proteins have attached themselves to specific components of the cell.

Third paragraph: cites an example—fluorescently labeled proteins.

Topic: This is an information passage on lenses in microscopes. You can certainly expect questions on lenses and maybe on fluorescence.

Now let's look at another example.

> The mass spectrometer is a device that utilizes electric and magnetic fields to determine the masses of the elements or compounds that exist within a certain sample. The operation of the mass spectrometer relies on the fact that the path of a moving charge is affected by the presence of electric and magnetic fields.

Coupled with the Figure, you can tell that this is an experiment passage—about a mass spectrometer. You'll need to read the experimental details carefully.

To analyze a sample, it must first be ionized. This may be accomplished by bombarding it with a stream of electrons. The ionized particles are then accelerated through a potential difference of several thousand volts that is set up between two slits S_1 and S_2 (see figure below). For the mass spectrometer to give useful results, all the particles entering the chamber below S_3 must be traveling at the same velocity. This is assured by passing the particles through a *velocity selector*, a region of a crossed magnetic field, B, and an electric field, E, located between S_2 and S_3. This electric field is produced by two charged parallel plates, P_1 and P_2. Only particles that are traveling at a velocity such that the force due to the electric field (qE) and that due to the magnetic field (qvB) cancel one another will remain undeflected and pass through the slit in S_3.

This paragraph provides the details of the experiment—underline and understand how it works. Only charged particles of a certain velocity pass through.

The stream of charged particles then pass though another magnetic field, B', but this time, there is no electric field. The second magnetic field is perpendicular to the page, and deflects the particles in a circular path, towards the detector. Based on the radius of curvature of the path of the particle, its mass can be determined from the formula:

$$\frac{q}{m} = \frac{E}{rBB'}$$

where q is the charge of the particle, m is the mass of the particle, E is the electric field, and r is the radius of the circular path of the particle. In the mass spectrometer below, $E = 8 \times 10^4$ V/m, $B = 0.4$ T, and $B' = 0.5$ T. The fundamental unit of charge is 1.6×10^{-19} C.

Second paragraph: What happens to the charges as they leave the velocity selector—mass is measured based on how curved their paths are in another magnetic field.

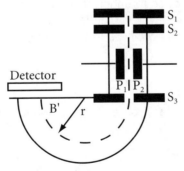

Figure 1 Mass Spectrometer

The Figure—can you see how the components of the setup contribute to the experiment?

Topic: An experiment passage, in which the masses of charged particles are measured using electric and magnetic fields. Expect questions on E-fields and on magnetism.

Could you, without looking back to the last passage, describe how the experiment is carried out? Unlike an Organic Chemistry passage, it's important in a Physics passage to read these portions carefully.

HANDLING THE QUESTIONS

There is certainly more than one method for handling questions, but at the foundation of each is the idea that the test taker's grounding in basic physics must be good. There are few "plug-and-chug" or graph interpretation–like questions in MCAT Physics. As you read in chapter 5, four types of questions appear in the science sections of the MCAT:

Discrete questions: These are the questions that don't accompany a passage; blocks of discrete questions are always preceded by a warning, such as "Questions 115 through 119 are NOT based on a descriptive passage." If you don't know the relevant science, you don't have much hope of getting these questions right. There isn't a passage to fall back on. All the information you'll need will be in the question stem, the answer choices, and your outside knowledge.

Questions that stand alone from the passage: These are questions that follow a passage, but for all practical purposes are discrete questions. Usually they are thematically related to the passage (for example, an unrelated question on photon energies might follow a passage about laser standing waves), but require no information from the passage. In Physics, you'll get a lot of questions of this type following an information passage.

Questions where you need only data from the passage: These questions can't be answered without the passage—but you don't need to understand the passage to do so. At best, all you'll need is data from the passage. You'll need only outside knowledge to figure out how to answer the question.

Questions that require an understanding of the passage: In Physics, you'll mostly find this type of question following experiment passages. This type of question can't be answered solely by applying outside knowledge; you'll need to understand at least a portion of the passage. Once you have read the passages the Kaplan way, you'll either have already absorbed from the passage the information you'll need, or know exactly where in the passage to go back and get it.

Answering the Questions

Following the steps outlined in chapter 5 on every question will help you develop habits that lead you to a higher score on Test Day.

Understand what you are being asked.

The first thing you want to do is to read the entire question, including the answer choices. Some MCAT science questions can seem very confusing as you read them. Reading the answer choices right after reading the question stem will help you focus on how to go about solving the problem. You can waste a lot of time trying to come up with the answer to a question you don't really understand.

Sometimes, the question will ask for something very directly. Consider this discrete question:

$$^{228}_{89}\text{Ac} \rightarrow {}^{228}_{90}\text{Th} + \text{X}$$

What decay particle does X represent?

    A.   Alpha particle

    B.   Gamma ray

    C.   Positive beta particle (positron)

    D.   Negative beta particle (electron)

You are asked to figure out what type of particle X is, given the parent and daughter nuclei.

There are times when you may read the question stem and still not quite understand what you need to do to get the right answer. This is why you should read the answer choices along with the question stem. The next example follows the mass spectrometer passage:

If the voltage at S_1 is 10,000 V, and at S_2 is zero V, how much work is done by the electric force on a doubly ionized particle between S_1 and S_2?

    A.   0 eV

    B.   5,000 eV

    C.   10,000 eV

    D.   20,000 eV

Since the answer choices are numbers, a *calculation* is required for the work due to an electric field.

A close relative of this question type is the question that asks you to remember the relevant formula, but doesn't require you to carry out the calculation. Always be careful to use the right units on questions like this. This example follows the microscope passage:

The objective has a focal length of 6.0 mm and is located at a distance of 6.2 mm from the specimen under consideration. How far away from the objective will the image be?

    A. $\dfrac{(6.0)(6.2)}{6.2 - 6.0}$ mm

    B. $\dfrac{6.2 - 6.0}{(6.0)(6.2)}$ mm

    C. $\dfrac{6.0 - 6.2}{(6.0)(6.2)}$ mm

    D. $\dfrac{(6.0)(6.0)}{6.2 - 6.0}$ mm

The answer choices are formulas, so no calculations are required, but you'll need to know the formula that gives you the image distance.

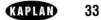

There will be times when the answer choices won't hint directly at what you need to do, but will instead put a limit on the number of things you'll have to think about. Consider the following question, which follows the microscope passage:

> Which of the following accurately describes the image formed by placing the object farther from the objective than the objective's focal point?
>
> A. The image is inverted and enlarged.
> B. The image is inverted and shrunk.
> C. The image is upright and enlarged.
> D. The image is upright and shrunk.

Even if you can't figure out whether the image is inverted or upright, but can determine whether it's enlarged or shrunk, you can at least eliminate two answer choices as wrong—and you've got a 50-50 shot at getting this question right.

It is not always so easy to decipher what the question is looking for. On many questions, you will need to translate or paraphrase the question stem. Rephrase the question, in your own words, paring it down to its essentials. To do this, you have to ask yourself, "What am I really being asked?" Perhaps you've heard the expression about being able to "see the forest for the trees." The questions on the MCAT can seem very daunting, so it's essential to take a step back, and connect what you see in the question to both the passage and the science concepts that might be involved in answering the question.

Answering the question, "What am I being asked?" can be particularly important for Physics questions. Difficult Physics questions are made difficult by obscuring the fact that you are being asked only to apply basic concepts from physics.

Consider this example, from the microscope passage:

> A bacterium is studied by using a microscope whose lens magnifies the specimen $100\times$ and whose eyepiece magnifies the specimen $10\times$. If the bacterium appears to be 2 mm long, what is the actual size of the bacterium?
>
> A. $2\ \mu m$
> B. $20\ \mu m$
> C. $0.5\ \mu m$
> D. $50\ \mu m$

The question that must be answered before you can calculate the actual size of the bacterium is: Given the magnification of each lens individually, what is the total magnification when both are used together? In this question, notice that it's the middle stage that the MCAT is really testing. If you were asked, "A 2-mm object has been magnified $1,000\times$. What is its actual size?" it wouldn't take you long to divide 2 mm by 1,000 and get the correct answer. What the MCAT wants to know is, "If we give the test taker the magnification of both lenses separately, will she or he know how to combine them and then calculate the correct answer?" You will be ready for these "questions behind the question" when you have mastered the Physics you've learned in class, and had lots of practice with MCAT-style passages.

One important note: *There isn't a magic wand that you can wave that makes all MCAT questions easy to answer.* The good news is, the concepts the MCAT tests are finite in number. As you practice Physics passages, you will see that some passages and questions are harder than others, requiring you to step back and determine what basic concepts the questions are *really* asking you to use.

Figure out where to go and get any information that you need.

Now that you understand what the question is asking for, you'll want to figure out what you are going to do to get to the correct answer. Normally, once you understand the question, your knowledge of the sciences will tell you exactly what's going on, and the path to the correct answer will be clear.

Where you will need to go to find any information you'll need will largely depend on the type of question. If you are tackling a discrete question, independent of any passages, the only place for you to look besides the question stem and the answer choices is to your brain—discrete questions always call upon outside science knowledge.

For questions that can stand alone from the passage, you'll need neither information from nor understanding of the passage. You'll have to rely on your outside knowledge again. Most of the questions following information passages will be of this variety. But how do you know whether or not a question relies on the passage? If you read the information passage for structure, to understand the gist of what was going on, then you'll probably be able to recognize when a question presents a new situation, a scenario that falls outside the discussion in the passage. For example, imagine this question following the microscope passage:

A converging lens has a focal length of 4 cm. What is the magnification of an image due to an object placed 3 cm away from the lens?

A. −12
B. −4
C. 1
D. 4

The topic of the passage was lenses in microscopes. This question gives information about a specific lens, and makes no reference whatsoever to the passage. This question calls upon your ability to remember how the object distance, image distance, and focal length of a converging lens relate to each other—you need nothing from the passage.

Some questions will require you to go back to the passage for information, but not for understanding. Usually, this means that to answer the question, you need to use data given in the passage. Consider this example from the mass spectrometer passage:

What is the force on a singly charged ion due to the electric field between plates P_1 and P_2?

    A. 6.4×10^{-20} N

    B. 8.0×10^{-20} N

    C. 8.0×10^{-15} N

    D. 1.3×10^{-14} N

The question asks you to calculate the force due to an electric field on a particle. You'll need to come up with the formula for the force on an electric charge in an electric field by yourself. You'll need the electric field strength and the charge on a singly charged ion—both provided by the passage.

Experiment passages will be followed mostly by questions requiring that you understand the passage in detail. This is why you need to read the passage so closely the first time. Look at this question from the mass spectrometer passage:

What is the velocity of particles entering the mass spectrometer?

    A.   q/m

    B.   E/B'

    C.   B'/E

    D.   E/B

This question requires that you understand how the mass spectrometer works—not a surprise, coming from an experiment passage. Indeed, the passage has something very detailed to say about the velocity of particles in the spectrometer: The velocity selector ensures that only particles with speeds such that the electric and magnetic forces on them are in balance will pass through.

If you hadn't read for the details of how the experiment was carried out, you would now have to spend a lot of time rereading the passage, to try to figure out how to calculate the velocity of the particles. Realistically, if you read the experimental details carefully, but didn't remember how the velocity selector works, then at least you'd know where exactly to go back and reread.

Integrating science knowledge with any necessary passage research, determine the correct answer.

This is where you pull it all together and come up with the answer. If you've managed to avoid needing any outside science knowledge, you'll probably need it now. This is when it's important to remember two things:

- If you are doing a calculation, always be sure that your units are correct and consistent.
- The MCAT isn't asking you to reinvent the field of physics. If you get stuck on a spring question, ask yourself, "What are all the things I know about springs?" You might surprise yourself with all the things you can come up with.

Let's have a look at how some of the problems you've seen in the past few pages finish up.

KAPLAN

If the voltage at S_1 is 10,000 V, and at S_2 is zero V, how much work is done by the electric force on a doubly ionized particle between S_1 and S_2?

   A.   0 eV

   B.   5,000 eV

   C.   10,000 eV

   D.   20,000 eV

Since the answer choices are numbers, a calculation is required for the work due to an electric field.

The reason the electron-volt (eV) is convenient as a unit is because one eV is the energy a singly ionized particle (q=e) loses as it travels across a one-volt potential. So, remembering that the work done on charge q in traveling through a potential difference V is W = qV, you can calculate:

W = (2e)(10000 V) = 20,000 eV, choice **D**.

What is the velocity of particles entering the mass spectrometer?

   A.   q/m

   B.   E/B'

   C.   B'/E

   D.   E/B

As we've seen before, this question requires that you understand how the mass spectrometer described in this experiment passage works. The passage tells us that the velocity selector ensures that only particles with speeds such that the electric and magnetic forces on them are in balance will pass through.

From our outside knowledge, you know that the force on a charge due to an electric field is qE, and the force by a magnetic field on a charge q moving at speed v is qvB. Since the velocity selector acts between S_2 and S_3, the correct magnetic field to use is B, not B' (eliminate choices **B** and **C**). So, since theses two forces balance for particles that traverse the spectrometer: qE = qvB, v = E/B, choice **D**.

Here's a completely new question, from the spectrometer passage.

The electric field points from the positive to the negative plate, or in other words, towards the right. What is the direction of the magnetic field B?

   A.   To the left

   B.   Into the page

   C.   Out of the page

   D.   It is unrelated to the direction of the electric field

The question asks for the direction of the magnetic field B, given that the electric field points from left to right. The real question here is, is there a relationship between the direction of E and the direction of B, or is choice **D** correct?

To answer that question, you need to understand how and why the spectrometer works. According to the second paragraph, the region of interest is called the velocity selector; in it, the E and B fields are crossed in such a way that the magnetic force on the charges traveling down the page tends to cancel the force due to the electric field. Since the field points to the right, the electric force on the charges is to the right. So the magnetic force must be to the left. Now you understand the real question: In what direction should B point so that the magnetic force on the charges is to the left?

You can use the right-hand rule to work it out. The fingers point in the direction of the velocity, to the right, and the thumb points towards the force, to the left. So the fingers, which point in the direction of the field, must curl upwards, out of the page. Choice **C** is correct.

What follows is a list of the physics skills and concepts that you should have mastered before taking the MCAT. If you find that you are weak in any of these areas, incorporate these concepts into your study schedule.

IN PREPARING FOR THE MCAT, I SHOULD UNDERSTAND...

1.   Kinematics

- The four fundamental physical dimensions and their SI units
- The difference between displacement and distance traveled
- The difference between velocity and speed
- The difference between instantaneous velocity and average velocity
- The difference between instantaneous acceleration and average acceleration
- How graphs of position, velocity and acceleration versus time relate to physical motion
- The equations for motion under constant acceleration, and when each is useful
- The types of initial conditions which occur in free fall, and how to use the equations for motion under constant acceleration appropriately

2.   Newtonian Mechanics

- What a force is and how it affects the object to which it is applied
- Newton's First Law and what it implies
- Newton's Second Law and what it implies
- How to construct force-body diagrams for objects experiencing external forces, and how to apply Newton's Second Law to those diagrams
- Newton's Third Law and what it implies
- The two types of friction and how each is applied
- Newton's Law of Gravitation and how it is applied
- How Newton's Second Law is affected by uniform circular motion
- What torque is and how it affects the object to which it is applied
- Translational equilibrium and rotational equilibrium, and the circumstances that cause each to occur.

 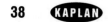

3.   Energy and Momentum

- The definition of work and how doing work affects the energy of an object
- The definition of kinetic energy
- The relationship between the net work done on an object and the object's kinetic energy
- The formulas for gravitational potential energy, in general and near the earth
- Under which circumstances the total mechanical energy of a system is conserved, and how to use the conservation of energy to solve problems
- The difference between conservative forces and nonconservative forces
- The concept of the average power applied to a system by having work done on it
- The definitions of the momentum of an object and the momentum of a system
- The conditions under which the total momentum of a system is conserved
- The differences among elastic, inelastic, and totally inelastic collisions, and what each implies about the system
- The definition of impulse, and the consequences of applying an average force to an object over a short period of time

4.   Thermodynamics

- What *temperature* means and the different temperature scales
- What *heat* is, and how it is different from temperature
- How materials expand and contract as their temperature changes
- All three parts of the first law of thermodynamics, and how the law is applied
- The definition of entropy
- How the second law of thermodynamics is applied, and the difference between the entropy of an object and the entropy of a system of objects

5.   Fluids and Solids

- The definition of density
- The definition of pressure
- The difference between gauge pressure and total pressure
- Pascal's principle and how it is applied
- The formula for hydrostatic pressure and how it is applied
- The formula for the buoyant force and how it is applied to Newton's second law
- The density rule and the definition of specific gravity
- How the continuity equation applies to a fluid
- How Bernoulli's equation applies to nonviscous fluids, and its common applications
- The definition of viscosity and how it affects other fluid concepts
- The definitions of stress and strain, and how they relate to Young's modulus and shear modulus; have a basic understanding of what Young's modulus means

6.   Electrostatics

- The definition of electric charge
- Coulomb's law and how different charges exert a force on one another

- What an electric field is and under what conditions it arises
- Electric field due to charge, and the difference between a test charge and a source charge
- The properties of electric field lines
- How to calculate the total electric field at one point due to multiple sources
- The effects on a conductor due to an external electric field
- The definition of electric potential energy and how it applies to systems of point charges
- The definition of electric potential, how electric potential is different than electric potential energy, and how electric potential is applied to point charges and parallel plates of opposite charge

7. DC/AC Circuits

- The definition of current, and conventional current
- The definition of direct current (DC)
- How an electromotive force (emf) isn't a force, but a potential difference, and how an emf generates current in a wire
- The definition of resistance
- Ohm's law, and how it applies not only to circuits as a whole, but also to individual circuit elements (resistors, charged capacitors, batteries)
- How resistors operate in series and in parallel in a circuit
- How the internal resistance of a battery can influence a circuit
- The definition of resistivity and how it is applied
- The function and properties of capacitors
- The definition of capacitance and how much energy can be stored in a capacitor
- How capacitors operate in series and in parallel in a circuit
- What a dielectric is, and how inserting a dielectric into a capacitor influences its properties
- How systems with current use power, and how much power is given off by a resistor due to heat
- What alternating current (AC) is, and why we measure root-mean-square (rms) voltages and currents

8. Magnetism

- What magnetic fields are, and how they are generated
- The formula for the magnetic field generated due to a current-carrying straight wire
- The formula for the magnetic field generated due to a current-carrying loop of wire
- The magnetic force law, and when an object experiences a force due to a magnetic field
- How to calculate the force on a charge in a magnetic field
- How to calculate the force on a current-carrying wire in an external magnetic field

9. Periodic Motion

- What simple harmonic motion is
- Hooke's law, and how to apply it using Newton's second law

 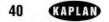

- How to calculate the frequency, angular frequency and period of a system undergoing simple harmonic oscillation
- How simple harmonic motion applies to springs
- How simple harmonic motion applies to pendula, as opposed to springs

10. Waves

- The properties of waves: speed, amplitude, intensity, and transverse or longitudinal oscillation
- Under what conditions two waves with the same frequency experience constructive and destructive interference, and what it means for two waves of the same frequency to be in phase, 90° out of phase, and 180° out of phase
- How the general properties of waves apply to sound waves, including the decibel scale, pitch, beat frequency, and the Doppler effect
- How standing waves are generated in oscillating systems of fixed length

11. Light and Optics

- The speed of light, and how it relates to frequency and wavelength
- What photons are
- How photons oscillate, what linear polarization is, and the effects of placing a polarizer in the path of a light wave
- The law of reflection
- The definition of *the index of refraction, Snell's law of refraction* and how to apply it
- The circumstances under which total internal reflection occurs
- The lens-makers equation, the sign conventions for object distance, image distance, and focal length, what magnification is and how to apply it, and how to treat light traveling through multiple lenses

12. Atomic Phenomena

- The phenomena of atomic electron energy levels, and how the binding energy depends on principal quantum number
- How electrons can transition between energy levels by emitting or absorbing photons

13. Nuclear Phenomena

- What the atomic number and mass number of a nucleus mean in terms of what's inside
- The relationship between rest mass and its equivalent energy
- Why the mass of a nucleus doesn't equal the sum of the masses of its parts
- That not all isotopes are stable, and that unstable nuclei undergo radioactive decay into other nuclei, the four common type of radioactive decay, and what the half-life of an unstable isotope is.

PHYSICS PRACTICE SET

Answer Sheet

1 Ⓐ Ⓑ Ⓒ Ⓓ   16 Ⓐ Ⓑ Ⓒ Ⓓ   31 Ⓐ Ⓑ Ⓒ Ⓓ

2 Ⓐ Ⓑ Ⓒ Ⓓ   17 Ⓐ Ⓑ Ⓒ Ⓓ   32 Ⓐ Ⓑ Ⓒ Ⓓ

3 Ⓐ Ⓑ Ⓒ Ⓓ   18 Ⓐ Ⓑ Ⓒ Ⓓ   33 Ⓐ Ⓑ Ⓒ Ⓓ

4 Ⓐ Ⓑ Ⓒ Ⓓ   19 Ⓐ Ⓑ Ⓒ Ⓓ   34 Ⓐ Ⓑ Ⓒ Ⓓ

5 Ⓐ Ⓑ Ⓒ Ⓓ   20 Ⓐ Ⓑ Ⓒ Ⓓ   35 Ⓐ Ⓑ Ⓒ Ⓓ

6 Ⓐ Ⓑ Ⓒ Ⓓ   21 Ⓐ Ⓑ Ⓒ Ⓓ   36 Ⓐ Ⓑ Ⓒ Ⓓ

7 Ⓐ Ⓑ Ⓒ Ⓓ   22 Ⓐ Ⓑ Ⓒ Ⓓ   37 Ⓐ Ⓑ Ⓒ Ⓓ

8 Ⓐ Ⓑ Ⓒ Ⓓ   23 Ⓐ Ⓑ Ⓒ Ⓓ   38 Ⓐ Ⓑ Ⓒ Ⓓ

9 Ⓐ Ⓑ Ⓒ Ⓓ   24 Ⓐ Ⓑ Ⓒ Ⓓ   39 Ⓐ Ⓑ Ⓒ Ⓓ

10 Ⓐ Ⓑ Ⓒ Ⓓ   25 Ⓐ Ⓑ Ⓒ Ⓓ   40 Ⓐ Ⓑ Ⓒ Ⓓ

11 Ⓐ Ⓑ Ⓒ Ⓓ   26 Ⓐ Ⓑ Ⓒ Ⓓ   41 Ⓐ Ⓑ Ⓒ Ⓓ

12 Ⓐ Ⓑ Ⓒ Ⓓ   27 Ⓐ Ⓑ Ⓒ Ⓓ   42 Ⓐ Ⓑ Ⓒ Ⓓ

13 Ⓐ Ⓑ Ⓒ Ⓓ   28 Ⓐ Ⓑ Ⓒ Ⓓ   43 Ⓐ Ⓑ Ⓒ Ⓓ

14 Ⓐ Ⓑ Ⓒ Ⓓ   29 Ⓐ Ⓑ Ⓒ Ⓓ   44 Ⓐ Ⓑ Ⓒ Ⓓ

15 Ⓐ Ⓑ Ⓒ Ⓓ   30 Ⓐ Ⓑ Ⓒ Ⓓ   45 Ⓐ Ⓑ Ⓒ Ⓓ

PHYSICS PRACTICE SET

Time: 60 Minutes—45 Questions

DIRECTIONS: There are seven passages and ten discrete questions in this physics test. Each passage is followed by five questions of above average difficulty. After reading a passage, select the one best answer to each question. If you are not certain of an answer, eliminate the alternatives that you know to be incorrect and then select an answer from the remaining alternatives.

Passage I (Questions 1–5)

The Hubble Space Telescope (HST) is an astronomical satellite in low orbit above Earth's atmosphere. The telescope provides the best photometric measurements ever to be achieved from any astronomical image.

Light enters the telescope and is focused by the primary mirror onto the secondary mirror. The secondary mirror then reflects light through a small hole in the primary mirror to the focal plane, which is shared by redirecting mirrors and electromagnetic measuring instruments. The redirecting mirrors send light to the guidance center and wide-field/planetary camera (Wiff-Pick). The rays of light that are not intercepted by the redirecting mirrors pass on to the instruments: The faint-object camera (FOC), the high-resolution spectrograph (HRS) and the faint-object spectrograph (FOS).

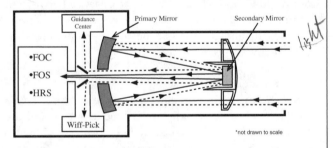

Figure 1

The primary mirror is approximately spherical and has a focal length of 58 m and a diameter of 2.4 m. The secondary mirror is flat and .3 m in diameter. The primary and secondary mirrors cooperatively focus the light at the focal plane. The mirrors are coated with aluminum and magnesium fluoride, giving them the capability to reflect light with wavelengths between 110 nm and 1 mm.

The HST enables astronomers to capture light from distant galaxies. Light emitted from the distant edges of the rapidly expanding universe is shifted to greater wavelengths by a quantity called the red shift (z):

$$z = \frac{\lambda_{obs} - \lambda_{emit}}{\lambda_{emit}}$$

Equation 1

where λ_{obs} is the wavelength of the light measured by the HST and λ_{emit} is the wavelength of the light emitted by the object.

The red shift is converted into R, the scale factor of the universe, using the formula:

$$R = \frac{1}{1 + z}$$

Equation 2

The value of R determines how large the universe was when it emitted the light. For example, if a galaxy is observed with a $z = 1$, then $R = 1/2$; the universe was one half its present size when the light was emitted.

[Note: $c = 3.00 \times 10^8$ m/s; $h = 6.626 \times 10^{-34}$ J·s]

1. Which of the following phenomena is responsible for the red shift?

   A. Ionization
   B. Reflection
   C. Refraction
   D. Doppler effect

GO ON TO THE NEXT PAGE.

2. Based on composition analysis, a certain star is expected to emit light with a wavelength of 250 nm. The FOS indicates that the star is emitting light with a wavelength of 750 nm. What was the relative size of the universe when the light was emitted?

A. 1/3

B. 1/2

C. 2

D. 3

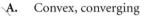

$\frac{750 - 250}{250} = \frac{500}{250} = 2$

$R = \frac{1}{1+2} = \frac{1}{3}$

3. The primary mirror can be described as

A. Convex, converging

B. Convex, diverging

C. Concave, converging

D. Concave, diverging

4. What are the radii of curvature of the primary and secondary mirrors respectively?

A. 1.2 m; 0.15 m

B. 29 m; 0.15 m

C. 29 m; infinity

D. 116m; infinity

5. If incoming parallel rays, when reflected by the mirrors, converge 2 m to the left of the reflective side of the primary mirror, what is the approximate distance between the two mirrors?

A. 14 m

B. 28 m

C. 58 m

D. 116 m

Passage II (Questions 6–10)

The Michelson interferometer exploits the phenomenon of interference between light waves. A simplified schematic of such a device is shown below:

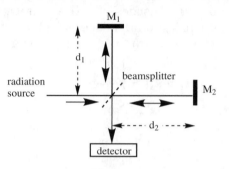

Figure 1

A beam of electromagnetic radiation (usually in either the visible or infrared region) falls upon a beamsplitter. The beamsplitter, which is essentially a mirror that is semitransparent to the radiation used, causes the beam of radiation to be split such that half of the intensity is transmitted while the other half is reflected. These two beams then strike mirrors M_1 and M_2, one of which is fixed and the other movable. The beams are reflected back towards the beamsplitter, where they interfere and are then directed towards the detector. In the diagram shown above, d_1 is the distance between the beamsplitter and M_1, and d_2 is the distance between the beamsplitter and M_2. Depending on the difference between d_1 and d_2, the two beams may interfere either constructively or destructively.

Consider the case where the radiation is monochromatic. If d_1 is equal to d_2, the distance traveled by the two beams of radiation will be identical, and thus the waves will interfere constructively. However, if the two distances differ by an amount x, the lengths of the paths traveled by the two beams will differ by $2x$. Destructive interference occurs when this difference of $2x$, known as the retardation, causes the two beams to be 180° out of phase.

As the movable mirror is translated, its distance from the beamsplitter increases smoothly, and so does the retardation. The intensity of the radiation reaching the detector will vary as the interference goes from constructive to destructive and back. The interferogram, a plot of the intensity versus retardation, will exhibit a sinusoidal shape: It will show a series of maxima and minima (bright and dark fringes) corresponding to constructive and destructive interferences, respectively

GO ON TO THE NEXT PAGE.

(Figure 2). The condition for constructive interference for the Michelson interferometer is:

$$|d_1 - d_2| = m\lambda/2$$

...where m = 0, 1, 2, … and λ is the wavelength of the radiation source.

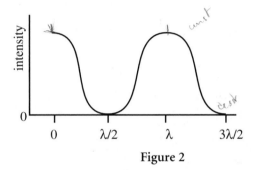

Figure 2

6. If a helium-neon laser is used as the light source (λ = 6328 Å), how far should the movable mirror be displaced to move from one bright fringe to the next one?

   A.   3164 Å
   B.   6328 Å
   C.   9492 Å
   D.   12660 Å

7. If the frequency of the monochromatic radiation is increased (all else being the same), which of the following would result?

     I. The maximum intensity registered by the detector would be lower.

     II. The minimum intensity registered by the detector would be lower.

     III. More maxima and minima will be encountered for a given distance.

   A.   I only
   B.   II only
   C.   III only
   D.   II and III only

8. If the source radiation consists of light of two distinct wavelengths λ_1 and λ_2 that are relatively close in value, which of the following characterizes the appearance of the interferogram?

   A.   A beat wavelength of $|\lambda_1 - \lambda_2|$
   B.   A beat wavelength of $|\lambda_1 + \lambda_2|$
   C.   A beat frequency of $\left|\dfrac{c}{\lambda_1} - \dfrac{c}{\lambda_2}\right|$
   D.   A beat frequency of $\left|\dfrac{c}{\lambda_1} + \dfrac{c}{\lambda_2}\right|$

9. One application of the interferometer is the determination of the index of refraction of a gas sample. If the wavelength of light in vacuum is λ_0, then how many wavelengths will fit in a distance d in a medium with an index of refraction of n?

   A. $n\lambda_0/d$
   B. nd/λ_0
   C. λ_0/nd
   D. $d/n\lambda_0$

10. If the source radiation consists of a continuous range of wavelengths, the resulting interferogram:

   A.   exhibits maximum constructive interference only when the retardation equals zero.
   B.   exhibits the same periodicity as the lowest wavelength component of the source radiation.
   C.   exhibits the same periodicity as the highest wavelength component of the source radiation.
   D.   exhibits no constructive interference.

GO ON TO THE NEXT PAGE.

Passage III (Questions 11–15)

A ship is engineered with the ability to right itself under severe environmental conditions. When waves and wind cause a ship to tilt, a torque is generated that restores the ship to equilibrium. However, if the angle of tilt is too great, a ship will overturn and sink.

On calm water, a ship is in rotational equilibrium. The forces of gravity and buoyancy act along the centerline of the ship and are equal in magnitude and opposite in direction. Figure 1 contains the major physical features of this system: The buoyant force (F_b) acts at the hydrostatic center (H), which is the center of gravity of the fluid displaced by the ship. The gravitational force (F_g) operates at the center of gravity of the ship (C). When a ship tilts, H shifts to the leaning side (the center of gravity does not shift) and the forces no longer operate along the same axis. The point at which the buoyant force vector intersects the centerline is called the metacenter (M). The displacement from C to M is called the metacentric height (m).

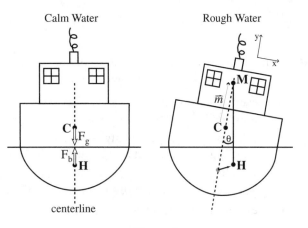

Figure 1

The buoyant force exerts a torque (τ) about the center of gravity according to the equation:

$$\tau = F_b m \sin \theta$$

Equation 1

...where F_b is the buoyant force, m is the metacentric height, and θ is the angle between the buoyant force vector and the metacentric height. The torque exerted by the buoyant force is referred to as the restoring torque.

The stability of the ship depends on the magnitude of the restoring torque. The restoring torque is proportional to the width of the ship, because the hydrostatic center gets displaced further away from the center line the farther the ship tilts. The restoring torque is inversely proportional to the height of the ship because the higher center of gravity decreases the metacentric height.

11. Which of the following is true as the ship tilts over?

      I. H is displaced further from the centerline

      II. A greater θ is created

      III. The buoyant force increases

  A.   I only

  B.   II only

  C.   I and II only

  D.   I, II and III

12. A ship will overturn when:

  A.   The force of gravity exceeds the buoyant force.

  B.   The metacentric height becomes negative.

  C.   The hydrostatic center and center of gravity do not lie in a vertical line.

  D.   The restoring torque reaches a minimum.

13. Which of the following correctly represents the mass of the water displaced by a tilting boat?

  A. $\dfrac{\tau}{F_b \sin \theta}$

  B. $\dfrac{\tau}{gm \sin \theta}$

  C. $\dfrac{F_b}{gV}$

  D. ρgV

14. According to Newton's third law, for every action there is an equal and opposite reaction. Which of the following is the reactive force to gravity on the ship?

  A.   The restoring torque

  B.   The buoyant force

  C.   The gravitational force on the earth due to the ship

  D.   The gravitational force on the fluid due to the ship

GO ON TO THE NEXT PAGE.

15. Which of the following represents the component of the buoyant force vector that generates the restoring torque?

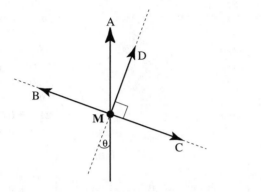

A. A

B. B

C. C

D. D

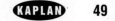

Passage IV (Questions 16–20)

A long plastic tube is partially filled with water as shown in Figure 1. A spigot at the bottom of the tube allows water to be drained away, lowering the water level.

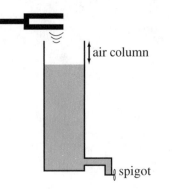

air column

spigot

Figure 1

A tuning fork of known frequency is struck with a rubber mallet and then placed near the open end of the tube, initiating vibrations of the air in the tube. The surface of the water always corresponds to a wave node and the mouth of the tube corresponds to an antinode.

While the tuning fork rings near the opening, the spigot is opened to lower the water level. This causes the length of the air column to increase, and occasionally it will reach a value at which the frequency of the fundamental, or one of its overtones, is the same as the frequency of the tuning fork (Figure 2). When this happens, resonance occurs and a loud ringing response is heard.

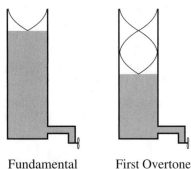

Fundamental   First Overtone

Figure 2

The values of the air column lengths corresponding to resonance are recorded below:

Frequency of tuning fork (Hz)	Length of air column at resonance (cm)
256	31.9 ± 0.5
	96.0 ± 0.5
426.7	20.0 ± 0.5
	59.8 ± 0.5
384	21.5 ± 0.5
	66.3 ± 0.5

Table 1

16. In the experiment, which of the following could be the next resonance value of the length of the air column, using the tuning fork of 426.7 Hz?

    A. 80 cm

    B. 100 cm

    C. 120 cm

    D. 160 cm

17. The speed of sound in air decreases as the temperature decreases. If the experiment were conducted at a lower temperature,

    A. the air column lengths at resonance would decrease.

    B. the air column lengths at resonance would increase.

    C. the frequency of the standing waves would decrease.

    D. the frequency of the standing waves would increase.

18. The experiment is performed again using a liquid other than water to partially fill the tube. The results of the experiment turn out to be the same as that recorded in Table 1. What can we conclude about that liquid?

    A. It has the same density as water.

    B. It has the same index of refraction as water.

    C. It has the same molecular weight as water.

    D. Its properties relative to water cannot be determined.

GO ON TO THE NEXT PAGE.

KAPLAN

CHAPTER FIVE

General Chemistry

We have already developed a repertoire of general strategies and methods to use with MCAT passages and questions. Now let's concentrate on the specifics of General Chemistry. General Chemistry passages and discrete questions appear as part of the Physical Sciences section of the MCAT, but they are not distinguished in any way from the Physics passages and questions. Therefore, it is up to you to determine which portions are General Chemistry–based, and apply our strategies accordingly.

One of the most difficult aspects of the MCAT is in reading the passages. Test takers tend to waste a lot of time reading passages the same way they read a textbook or a newspaper; they attempt to understand completely every argument made and every detail given. While useful for a history or biology test, this type of reading will not pay off on Test Day. The MCAT science passages are full of data that will always be there if you need it. When you read a passage, take a broad look at what is happening and think about what basic science concepts are being applied in the situations described in the passage. Allow yourself a maximum of 60 seconds to absorb what you need from the passage. In this chapter, you will practice reading General Chemistry passages quickly, going into the questions having a good sense of the passage, and being prepared for what may arise. Included in your arsenal of General Chemistry skills for Test Day should be those listed later on in this chapter. Excelling in General Chemistry on the MCAT depends in part on mastery of this skill set.

READING THE PASSAGE

Passage Types

General Chemistry passages fall into the three categories described in chapter 5, but are also unique in many ways.

Information passages read very much like textbooks or scientific review journals and usually explain the chemistry behind some natural phenomenon. In General Chemistry, these passages are very graphics-intensive, so you should expect to see reactions, equations, tables, or graphs.

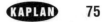

The text functions primarily to explain the graphics and put them in some sort of context.

Experiment passages typically consist of brief background information about some compound, reaction, or chemical process, followed by a series of experiments and a presentation of results. These passages read very much like laboratory manuals or reports. The purpose of the experiments is usually stated in the first sentence of the passage. Numerical results may be presented in a table or graph.

Persuasive argument passages present contrasting views on a subject. The typical format is for the passage to introduce a chemical phenomenon, and then present the differing viewpoints as hypotheses. Many of the questions will then rely on understanding the similarities and the differences of the hypotheses. Since persuasive argument passages are rare in the General Chemistry portion of the MCAT, you can focus primarily upon information and experiment passages.

Mapping the Passage

As you learned in chapter 5, passage mapping is the process by which you create a "map" of the main ideas and critical concepts. Mapping is the best way to grasp the structure of a passage without getting bogged down or confused by detail. In General Chemistry, mapping a passage consists of two steps: Mapping graphics and mapping text.

Mapping Graphics

A surprisingly high percentage of General Chemistry questions can actually be answered using only the graphics found in a passage. In General Chemistry passages, you will encounter five types of graphics: Graphs, tables, reactions, equations, and figures. If a graphic exists in a passage, you are likely to be asked about it.

>*Graphs and Tables*: Graphs typically present the results of some experiment or series of measurements. Tables may often do the same, but can also show you the physical or chemical properties of some element or compound. When mapping a graph or table, you should primarily be noting:
>
>- The subject of the graphic
>- Any obvious trends or similarities
>
>Frequently the subject of the graphic will be explicitly stated in the caption—it is simply what the graphic presents to you (e.g., the dissociation constants for several compounds). You should make some quick and obvious deductions from the graphic. If a table displays the results of some experiment, you may want to figure out what the results show you. Below you will find an example of a table that you might find on the MCAT. The types of observations recorded beside the table are similar to those you should be making as you map the passage.

Table 1 Electron Affinities of Several Elements

Element	Electron Affinity (eV)
Li	0.618
H	0.754
C	1.26
O	1.46
Br	3.36
F	3.40

Subject: electron affinities of several elements. There's nothing new here—just specific values that reflect trends you should already know.

You should be sure to note the subject of the table/graph in the margins. This will help you find information when you refer back to the passage to answer questions. Other observations and deductions should probably be made only in your head, since they may take longer to write down. If a graph or table does not demand obvious interpretation, then don't waste time looking for one. Remember that the MCAT only rewards you for correctly answering questions, not understanding passages.

Reactions: Mapping an equation or reaction should be done with a more focused approach than with a graph, table, or figure, since you know the range of General Chemistry reaction types possible on the MCAT. Questions you should be asking yourself when you see an equation include:

- What is the reaction type: acid-base, redox, or other?
- What are the species involved?
- Are there phases or phase changes?
- Is the reaction in equilibrium, or does it run to completion?

This list is neither exhaustive nor rigid. With practice you will see that these kinds of observations will help you better understand passages without wasting time on unnecessary detail.

When you are shown a series of reactions, you should also pay attention to how they are most obviously related—again, looking for trends and similarities. For example, if you are given three equations, and ammonia shows up in all three, it is likely that the text of the passage talks about different reactions of ammonia. Similarly, if you are given four acid-base reactions, you should expect to see some acid-base questions. However, you should NOT sit and brainstorm possible question types on test day. The questions are right there on the next column or page—go ahead and answer them!

Let's look at the example below and see what we can learn from the equations given:

Step 1: $Cl_2 \rightarrow 2\ Cl\bullet$
Step 2: $Cl\bullet + CH_4 \rightarrow CH_3 + HCl$
Step 3: $CH_3 + Cl_2 \rightarrow CH_3Cl + Cl\bullet$
Step 4: $Cl\bullet + CH_3\bullet \rightarrow CH_3Cl$

Your notes might read:

4-step radical chain rxn
$Cl\bullet$ not consumed
$Cl_2 + CH_4 \rightarrow CH_3Cl$

Mapping Text

After you have mapped the graphics found within the passage, your next step is to map the text. As previously stated, you shouldn't read a passage trying to memorize every detail. Instead, you should employ your critical reasoning skills. You want to come out of each paragraph having gotten the gist of what's going on. As you finish each paragraph, ask, "What is this paragraph doing?" Make note of the main ideas and major concepts of the text so that you can find the details later, if needed. The extent to which you annotate as you read a passage depends upon your individual comfort level. As you begin to practice reading passages, annotate them, and then wean yourself off of written notes as you become more and more comfortable keeping the necessary information in your head. As you annotate, be sure to summarize each paragraph, underlining the meanings of new terms or equations.

The degree of detail you need to absorb from the text depends on the type of passage. Information passages are filled with text that is primarily complementary to the equations/tables presented. The important information in these passages can be almost entirely discerned from the graphics, so skim the text very quickly. You need to know only what the text is about, not what it actually says. Experiment passages, on the other hand, are more conceptually difficult, and require you to follow the logical progression of some experiment. After an experiment passage, there is likely to be at least one question asked that depends upon a detailed understanding of how the experiment works and what is being tested. You will want to read these passages with a much more critical mind than you would with an information passage. The same is true for persuasive argument passages, which can often be followed by a question or two that is tightly focused on one or more of the hypotheses.

Identifying the Topic

In addition to mapping the passage, you should also aim to *identify the topic* of the passage. This means more than simply coming up with a scientific term corresponding to the main subject of the passage. Rather, identifying the topic means answering the question, "What is the author trying to do in the passage?" Being able to answer this question means that you have read the passage critically—and critical reading is the most important skill for reading MCAT passages.

Now that you've broken down the components of your passage-reading strategy, put them together and see how you might read a passage on Test Day. Look at the following information passage. It has been mapped using the techniques described on the previous pages. Although there is no one correct way to map a passage, the notes and observations written below the passage are similar to those you should be making on Test Day.

The concentration of <u>nitrogen oxides in our atmosphere</u> has greatly increased during the past century, having significant negative impact on the environment. Nitrous oxide (N_2O), which is released into the air by fertilizers and from newly cleared soil, is thought to contribute to the greenhouse effect by absorbing infrared radiation given off by the earth. Nitric oxide (NO) and nitrogen dioxide (NO_2) produced by the burning of organic material contribute to the phenomenon known as photochemical smog. Although smog is generally thought of as resulting from the burning of fossil fuels, the burning of vegetation in the tropics is also a source of air pollution.

Prose about NO_x sources.

On a smoggy day, the nitric oxide concentration in the air peaks early in the morning. This NO later combines with oxygen to form NO_2, which in turn combines with oxygen in a light-catalyzed reaction to form ozone (O_3).

Reaction 1: $2NO(g) + O_2(g) \rightarrow 2NO_2(g)$
$H° = -113$ kJ/mol $G° = -69.8$ kJ/mol
Reaction 2: $2NO_2(g) + O_2(g) \xrightarrow{hv} NO(g) + O_3(g)$
$H° = -199$ kJ/mol $G° = 298.3$ kJ/mol

rxns. and thermo. data for ozone formation

<u>Photochemical smog</u> attacks living matter such as plants and lung tissue; it also reacts with organic materials such as rubber and various atmospheric hydrocarbons. It reacts with moisture to form nitric acid, which corrodes metals and contributes to acid rain.

prose about effects of photochem. smog

To decrease smog levels, cars are equipped with <u>catalytic converters</u>, in which the following reactions take place.

Reaction 3: $2NO_2(g) \rightarrow 2O_2(g)$
$H° = -68$ kJ/mol $G° = -104$ kJ/mol
Reaction 4: $2NO(g) \rightarrow N_2 + O_2(g)$
$H° = -181$ kJ/mol $G° = -173$ kJ/mol
Reaction 5: $2NO + 2CO(g) \rightarrow 2CO_2(g) + N_2(g)$
$H° = -747$ kJ/mol $G° = -688$ kJ/mol
Reaction 6: $2NO(g) + 2H_2(g) \rightarrow 2H_2O(g) + N_2(g)$
$H° = -752$ kJ/mol $G° = -648$ kJ/mol

rxns. and thermo. data for breakdown of NO_x in catalytic converter

topic: discusses rxns. that break down atmospheric nitrogen oxides

This passage should not take you very long to map. The critical points are the two series of reactions and the thermodynamic data. From inspection, Reactions 1 and 2 show the formation of ozone (O_3). Reactions 3–6 involve nitrogen oxides, so the passage is about smog formation and decomposition. You should expect to answer questions about the thermodynamics of these processes.

Now let's see how a map for an experiment passage might look.

A chemist studies the thermodynamics of the equilibrium between SO_2, O_2, and SO_3. SO_2 and O_2 react to form SO_3 by the stoichiometric relationship given in Reaction 1.

$$2SO_2(g) + O_2(g) \rightleftarrows 2SO_3(g)$$

Reaction 1

rxn. being studied: gas-phase equilibrium

Sulfur dioxide and oxygen gas, at 298 K and 1 atm, are injected into an evacuated metal cylinder in a 2:1 molar ratio. The cylinder is then sealed so that the gases cannot escape. The chemist proceeds to heat the cylinder, pausing every 100 K. At each pause, the chemist measures the internal pressure after it has stabilized for at least twenty minutes. The table below shows the pressures recorded for a series of temperatures, as well as the pressures expected were the gases not to react.

experiment: measure pressure inside canister as function of temperature

Table 1 Total Internal Pressure at Various Temperatures

T (K)	P_r (P recorded after reaction, in atm.)	P_e (P expected without reaction, in atm.)
600	1.3	2.0
700	1.6	2.3
800	1.9	2.7
900	2.3	3.0
1000	2.8	3.3
1100	3.3	3.7
1200	3.8	4.0
1300	4.2	4.3

results: actual pressure gets closer to predicted pressure as temperature increases

topic: experiment about effect of temperature on reaction equilibrium

Again, you should not take more than 60 seconds to map a passage like this. This passage basically consists of one experiment studying the thermochemistry of one reaction. Though you should read the second paragraph closely enough that you understand how the experiment studies the thermodynamics of the reaction, the key elements of the passage are the reaction and the data table.

HANDLING THE QUESTIONS

Now that we've discussed how to read General Chemistry passages, let's move on to handling questions—the part of the test where you actually earn your points.

As you learned in chapter 5, you will encounter four types of MCAT science questions:

- *Discrete questions*
- *Questions that require an understanding of the passage*
- *Questions where you need only data from the passage*
- *Questions that can stand alone from the passage*

Discrete questions: These questions do not follow any passage and are always preceded by a warning such as "Questions 164 through 168 are NOT based on a descriptive passage." Consequently, all the information needed to answer these questions will be found in the question stem, the answer choices, and outside knowledge.

Questions that require an understanding of the passage: As opposed to discrete questions, these questions follow a passage and cannot be answered without having read the passage. These questions typically follow experiment or persuasive argument passages and less frequently, information passages (another reason why information passages should be read quickly). A question might ask you to interpret an experiment or a chemical process, and require that you have a conceptual understanding of topics discussed in the passage. For example, it would be difficult to answer the following question if you had not closely read the corresponding passage.

The gas that evolved when the chemist tried to dissolve element X was most likely:

- **A.** water vapor produced from the heat of reaction.
- **B.** oxygen produced by chemical reaction.
- **C.** hydrogen produced by chemical reaction.
- **D.** nitrogen that had been dissolved in the water from air.

Questions where you need only data from the passage: These questions are similar to the previous question type in that they cannot be answered without the passage. However, these questions do not demand a thorough understanding of the passage. Rather, they ask you to return to the passage to look at a table or equation—information that can be extracted from the passage without an understanding of their context or relevance. For example, a question might ask you to apply LeChatelier's principle to an equilibrium reaction found in the passage. In this case you do not need to know the relevance of that reaction; you just need to know what the reaction is so that you can apply your outside knowledge of LeChatelier's principle. Now let's take a look at the following question:

What is the rate law for Reaction 1?

- **A.** Rate $= k[NO_2]^2$
- **B.** Rate $= k[NO_2]^2[O_2]$
- **C.** Rate $= k[NO_2]^2[O_2][NO_2]^2$
- **D.** The rate of the reaction cannot be determined without more information.

All you need to answer this question is the stoichiometry of the reaction and/or some rate measurements. You don't need to understand the relevance of the reaction in context of the rest of the passage; in a case like this, you would just need to flip back to the passage to see what the reaction was.

Indeed, most General Chemistry questions on the MCAT can be answered using only pieces of information from the passage—an equation, a number, etc. Many, however, lead you to believe that you need a greater understanding of the passage than you actually do. These questions refer to compounds or reactions that are specific to the passage, tempting you to lean heavily on the passage for support. Still, the only information you need to retrieve from the passage for these questions is a number or a reaction—combing the passage for "the answer" will only waste time better spent thinking or checking answers. Most MCAT passages are filled with extraneous information that won't help you answer the questions. So when you refer back to a passage, do so with a very focused eye, looking only for the information specified by the questions.

Questions that can stand alone from the passage: These questions follow passages, but are in all other ways discrete questions. They require absolutely no knowledge or information from the passage, because they are related to the passage only in subject. The following question, for example, could follow the information passage that you read earlier about nitrogen oxide gases in our atmosphere.

What is the relationship between ΔG, ΔS, ΔH, and T?

    A. $\Delta G = \Delta S - T\Delta H$

    B. $\Delta G = T(\Delta H - \Delta S)$

    C. $\Delta G = \Delta H + T\Delta S$

    D. $\Delta G = \Delta H - T\Delta S$

Though linked to the passage by the subject of thermochemistry, the question can be solved using only our previous outside knowledge.

Determining the passage type will allow you to predict the types of questions you will see. Rarely will you need to return to an information passage to learn some logical sequence: You will usually return just to target specific kernels of information. Experiment and persuasive argument passages, on the other hand, are commonly followed by questions asking you to interpret experiments or hypotheses.

Answering the Questions

Correctly answering MCAT questions is highly correlated to efficiently identifying the essential underlying question and relevant science. The MCAT is designed to test our scientific thinking: Our ability to identify specific chemistry topics and apply them in new situations. So to become a better test taker, you need to look past the distraction of unfamiliar subjects and language, and look toward the core science of the question.

Understand what you are being asked.

The first thing to do is to read the question stem and the answer choices. Often, MCAT science questions can be confusing. Reading the answer choices after you read the question stem will help focus your thinking and provide useful clues. In this step, your goal is to boil down the question down to its essence and determine as precisely as possible what science concepts you're being asked about. You're not going to look back to the passage with a hazy notion of the question, hoping that something in the passage will suddenly crystallize your thinking. You need to know as precisely as possible the question being asked and the major chemistry concepts being tested, as illustrated by the following questions:

What factors directly contribute to the <u>average velocity</u> of gas particles?

I. Molecular mass

II. Temperature

III. Pressure

A. I and II only

B. I and III only

C. II and III only

D. I, II, and III

You are asked to identify those physical properties that directly affect gas particle velocity. Consider only molecular mass, temperature, and pressure.

Let's look at our next question:

What is the <u>rate law</u> for Reaction 1?

A. Rate $= k[NO_2]^2$

B. Rate $= k[NO_2]^2[O_2]$

C. Rate $= k[NO_2]^2[O_2][NO_2]^2$

D. The rate of the reaction cannot be determined without more information.

You are asked to determine the rate law for a reaction given in the passage. Reaction stoichiometry and rate measurements would be helpful.

Often, the question stem presents the science problem in a straightforward manner, in which case there is not much to do for this step.

What is the relationship between ΔG, ΔS, ΔH, and T?

A. $\Delta G = \Delta S - T\Delta H$

B. $\Delta G = T(\Delta H - \Delta S)$

C. $\Delta G = \Delta H + T\Delta S$

D. $\Delta G = \Delta H - T\Delta S$

You are asked to identify the mathematical relationship between four thermodynamic values.

However, sometimes the question stem may include unfamiliar language or bulky clauses. If this is the case, you'll paraphrase or translate the question stem in your mind, then look to the answer choices for additional hints.

If the KHP had been exposed to moisture prior to the titration, the calculated concentration of the $KOH(aq)$ would be:

Question: How does water affect the calculated titration measurement?

    A.   greater than the actual concentration, since the quantity of KHP actually titrated would be greater than the quantity used in calculations.

    B.   greater than the actual concentration, since the quantity of KHP actually titrated would be less than the quantity used in calculations.

    C.   less than the actual concentration, since the quantity of KHP actually titrated would be greater than the quantity used in calculations.

    D.   equal to the actual concentration, since the titration calculation depends on moles of KHP, not concentration.

You are asked to determine the effect of contaminants on titration points. You need to know what a titration measures and how it does that. Hint: Would you have to use more or less KHP to reach endpoint of titration, if KHP contains water?

If the question requires conceptual understanding of the passage, try to figure out what sorts of properties, relationships, or concepts you will be looking for.

Figure out where to go to get any information you may need.

Having a grasp of the problem at hand, use your passage map and science skill set to determine what information—both factual and conceptual—you may need to answer the question. Is the question topic something you should know? Does the question test a concept you should understand? (e.g., LeChatelier's principle, galvanic cells, etc.) Will concepts introduced in the passage help you? Do you need to retrieve facts from the passage (e.g., a value from a table or a compound from a reaction)? Using your passage map, figure out where this information is located. Below you will see how this step can be applied to the questions just covered.

What factors directly contribute to the average velocity of gas particles?

    I. Molecular mass

    II. Temperature

    III. Pressure

    A.   I and II only

    B.   I and III only

    C.   II and III only

    D.   I, II, and III

Pure outside knowledge: nothing is needed from the passage.

What is the rate law for Reaction 1?

A. Rate $= k[NO_2]^2$

B. Rate $= k[NO_2]^2[O_2]$

C. Rate $= k[NO_2]^2[O_2][NO_2]^2$

D. The rate of the reaction cannot be determined without more information.

Look at Reaction 1 and observe the stoichiometry. If reaction rate tables exist, look at them. If reaction rate is discussed in the passage, look at that text as well.

What is the relationship between ΔG, ΔS, ΔH, and T?

A. $\Delta G = \Delta S - T\Delta H$

B. $\Delta G = T(\Delta H - \Delta S)$

C. $\Delta G = \Delta H + T\Delta S$

D. $\Delta G = \Delta H - T\Delta S$

Pure outside knowledge: nothing is needed from the passage.

In the second example, the question stem does a pretty good job of telling you what information you need and where to find it. In the first and third examples, you recognized that the questions could be answered without returning to the passage. Being able to make such a determination requires a solid foundation in the science content, as well as a good passage map, which will give you a good sense of whether or not the passage will be of any help to you. A key part of learning science skills is not just being able to apply them when asked, but being able to identify when you need to use them. In the KHP question you saw earlier, you need to raise your level of critical thinking a bit to target what information will be useful.

If the KHP had been exposed to moisture prior to the titration, the calculated concentration of the KOH(aq) would be:

A. greater than the actual concentration, since the quantity of KHP actually titrated would be greater than the quantity used in calculations.

B. greater than the actual concentration, since the quantity of KHP actually titrated would be less than the quantity used in calculations.

C. less than the actual concentration, since the quantity of KHP actually titrated would be greater than the quantity used in calculations.

D. equal to the actual concentration, since the titration calculation depends on moles of KHP, not concentration.

You would want to refer back to the passage to find the titration reaction, as well as information on how the titration was performed.

Integrating science knowledge with any necessary passage research, determine the correct answer.

This last step is easier said than done. Here you will bring all components together: Outside knowledge, information from the passage, and reasoning/calculation. The exercises outlined in the last three steps should lead you to the content wall, the point at which getting the correct answer depends on scientific knowledge and reasoning skills.

Remember, test strategy is designed to complement, not replace your knowledge of MCAT General Chemistry. If you don't know the science, then there is little else you can do to improve your score. However, if you do have a grasp on the science, then adhering to solid test strategy will lead to points on Test Day.

Now let's take a look at our question strategy in action. The following questions, which pertain to the information passage about atmospheric nitrogen oxides you read earlier, have already been attacked using the method described above. Note how this method allows you to address more directly the basic science.

> What <u>reactions</u> would <u>occur spontaneously</u> under standard conditions?
>
> **A.** All except 2
> **B.** Only 2
> **C.** All except 5 and 6
> **D.** Only 1, 3, and 4

Q: How can you tell whether a reaction proceeds spontaneously? Look back to specific reactions (1–6) in the passage.

From the passage map you know you have six reactions, all with given values of H° and G°. If you remember that reaction spontaneity is related to some thermodynamic values, but don't know how, you could at least improve your chances of guessing correctly by noticing that Reaction 2 has thermodynamic values of opposite sign than the others. This reasoning would eliminate choices **C** and **D**. However, to answer correctly you must be able to recall that reactions proceed spontaneously when the Gibbs free energy has a negative value; the answer is therefore choice **A**.

> What values are commonly used to estimate enthalpies?
>
> **A.** Heat capacities
> **B.** Bond dissociation energies
> **C.** Oxidation states
> **D.** Activation energies

Q: What does enthalpy measure? How does enthalpy relate to what each value in the answer choices measures?

This question requires absolutely no information from the passage and is asked in a very straightforward manner. Without the passage, you should already know what enthalpy is and what the four answer choices measure. If you lack this knowledge, all you can do strategically is to eliminate those answers you know to be incorrect. The enthalpy of reaction is related to changes in energy associated with bond breaking and forming. The correct answer is therefore choice **B**.

Now, as an additional exercise, let's see how far we can progress with a series of questions given only the map of the passage upon which they are based.

Topic: discusses antacids and the regulation of stomach pH
- Prose regarding stomach biology
- Prose regarding antacids

Reaction: $Al(OH)_3 + 3HCl \rightarrow AlCl_3 + 3H_2O$

This passage is then followed by the following four questions:

How many grams of $AlCl_3$ are produced when 3 grams of $Al(OH)_3$ react completely with excess HCl?

A. 2.36 g

B. 3.00 g

C. 5.05 g

D. 9.07 g

How to handle this question: You are asked to calculate mass of reaction product; use stoichiometry skills. Your notes might read:

Q: 3g $Al(OH)_3$ + excess HCl → ? $AlCl_3$

How do you convert between mass and moles?

Reaction equation given in map includes all three species.

The basic question here is, "what is the stoichiometric relationship between $AlCl_3$ and $Al(OH)_3$?" Though this relationship is not something you would know off the top of your head, it can be found in the balanced equation given in the passage summary. You don't need to understand stomach acid, antacids, or the anything else from the passage: All the information you need can be extracted from the passage map, the periodic table (included at the front of your test booklet), and your outside knowledge.

If HCl is the only substance present in the stomach, what is the pH?

A. $-\log (0.15)$

B. $-\log (0.2)$

C. $\log (0.15)$

D. $\log (0.2)$

How to handle this question: You are asked to calculate the pH using acid concentration.

What is the relationship between pH and concentration?

How much HCl is there in the stomach? The prose about stomach biology may provide this info.

This question asks for the stomach pH, limiting your consideration to the effects of HCl. What do you know about HCl? Well, it's a strong acid, so it will dissociate completely in solution. Okay, so how much of it is in the stomach? This you probably don't know, so you look to the passage summary, which tells you that there is prose in the passage describing stomach biology. If indeed you were to refer to the passage, you could very quickly find that the concentration of HCl in the stomach is 0.15 N. With this little kernel of knowledge, you can now answer the question. 0.15 N HCl corresponds to a proton concentration of 0.15 M, since HCl is a strong monoprotic acid that will completely dissociate in solution. From our studies of acids and bases, you should recall that pH is related to the concentration of protons by pH = $-\log [H^+]$. Therefore the pH in the stomach is equal to $-\log (0.15)$, choice **A**.

While the active ingredients in most <u>antacids</u> are soluble in the acidic environment of the stomach, their <u>solubility is significantly reduced in pure water</u>. If a finely divided powder of one such compound, say $CaCO_3$, is mixed with deionized water, which of the following will be true?

You are asked to apply your knowledge of solution chemistry. Q: What happens when $CaCO_3$ is mixed with deionized water?

      I. The mixture will be homogeneous.

      II. A colloidal mixture will be formed.

      III. Separation of the mixture will produce a nonelectrolytic aqueous phase.

    A.   I only

    B.   III only

    C.   I and II only

    D.   II only

What is a colloidal mixture? What will the aqueous phase consist of?

The question stem here is very lengthy, but it provides you with all the information you need to answer the question. You are first told that antacids are not very soluble in pure water. You are then told that $CaCO_3$, an antacid, is mixed with deionized water. So what do you expect to happen? You should expect $CaCO_3$ will not dissolve in the water. With this expectation in mind, you are now ready to evaluate the three statements given to you. Statement I: Is the mixture of water and undissolved $CaCO_3$ homogeneous? No—there's a solid phase and a liquid phase. Eliminate choices **A** and **C**. Statement II: Is the mixture of water and undissolved $CaCO_3$ a colloid? Yes. Being able to recognize this depends on two sources of information: Your outside knowledge of what a colloid is and the statement in the question stem that the $CaCO_3$ is divided into a fine powder. Fine powders of insoluble substances become suspended in the liquid, forming a colloid. Choice **D** is correct. Statement III is false, since the aqueous phase contains no electrolytes; the only possible source of ions, $CaCO_3$, never entered the aqueous phase.

Strong, soluble bases such as alkaline earth metal hydroxides are not used as antacids, but are often used in laboratory titrations. What volume of an aqueous 1.5 M $Ba(OH)_2$ solution would be required to neutralize 10 mL of stomach acid?

You are asked to calculate the volume of base necessary to neutralize acid.

    A.   0.5 mL

    B.   1.5 mL

    C.   10.0 mL

    D.   15.0 mL

How many equivalents of protons are there in 10 mL of stomach acid? This is yet another question that can be answered using only tiny bits of information from the passage. Here, the task is relatively straightforward: You are to calculate the volume of a base of known strength that is sufficient to neutralize a known volume of an acid of known strength. The acid is again stomach acid, 0.15 N HCl. In 10 mL of stomach acid, there are 10 mL $\times$ (1 L / 1000 mL) $\times$ (0.15 mol H^+ / 1 L) = 1.5×10^{-3} mol H^+. To neutralize the acid, you need equal quantities of H^+ and OH^-. Each mole of the base, $Ba(OH)_2$, can give up two moles of hydroxide ions upon dissociation, and so a 1.5 M solution of the base has a normality of 3.0 N. The volume of the base you need to add is then (1.5×10^{-3} mol OH^-) / (3.0 mol OH^- / L) = 0.5×10^{-3} L = 0.5 mL, choice **A**.

A list of chemistry skills and concepts that you will need to have in your arsenal before taking the MCAT follows.

IN PREPARING FOR THE MCAT, I SHOULD UNDERSTAND...

1.   Atomic Structure / Periodic Table

- How to determine the electronic configurations of atoms/ions
- Periodic trends: atomic radii, ionization energy, electronegativity, electron affinity
- The four quantum numbers: how they are related and what each defines
- The chemical properties of groups
- Atomic absorption/emission and how to calculate photon energies

2.   Bonding

- Intermolecular forces: dipole-dipole, dispersion, and H-bonding
- Molecular/electronic geometry
- Resonance structures
- How to calculate formal charges
- Lewis structures
- Dipole moment, polarity, and their effects on reactivity
- The relation between bond length and bond energy

3.   Stoichiometry

- How to calculate the molecular weight of a compound
- How to balance a chemical equation
- How to calculate molecular composition by percent mass
- How molecular and empirical formulas are related
- Basic reaction types: single/double displacement, combustion, decomposition
- Limiting reagents and how to calculate percent yields

4. ## Kinetics / Rate Processes / Equilibrium
- Rate laws and reaction rate order
- LeChatelier's principle
- Energy profiles of reactions
- Chemical equilibrium, equilibrium constants, and law of mass action
- Catalysts

5. ## Thermochemistry
- Enthalpy: exothermic/endothermic
- State functions and thermodynamic terms (e.g., adiabatic, isobaric, etc.)
- How to calculate enthalpy changes of chemical processes (e.g., heat of vaporization, heat of reaction, etc.)
- Heat transfer and specific heat (calorimetry)
- Reaction profiles
- $\Delta G = \Delta H - T\Delta S$
- First law of thermodynamics: $\Delta E = Q - W$
- Gibb's free energy and spontaneity

6. ## Gases
- Kinetic molecular theory and its assumptions
- How to calculate average and root-mean-square molecular speeds, and rates of effusion and diffusion
- The ideal gas law, including Boyle's and Charles' laws
- How to calculate density and molar mass
- Van der Waals' equation of state

7. ## Phase Changes / Phase Equilibria
- Single and multiple component phase diagrams
- How to calculate colligative properties: vapor pressure lowering, boiling point elevation, freezing point depression, and osmotic pressure
- Phase equilibria and phase properties

8. ## Solutions
- Common ions by name, formula, and charge
- How to calculate ion concentration using K_{sp}, or vice versa
- How to calculate solution concentration: mole fraction, molarity, molality, normality, solution composition by percent mass
- The common ion effect

9. Acids and Bases

- How to identify Arrhenius/Bronsted/Lewis acids and bases
- How to identify conjugate acid-base pairs
- The conversion between p-scale and concentration/equilibrium constant
- How to interpret titration curves
- Strong acids/bases and weak acids/bases
- How to calculate pH of weak acid/base solutions
- Neutralization reactions and hydrolysis
- Amphoteric species and polyprotic acids
- Henderson-Hasselbalch equation

10. Electrochemistry

- The difference between electrolytic and galvanic cells and how it affects the designation of the cathode, anode, reduction electrode, oxidation electrode, electrode charge, electron flow, and ion flow in electrochemical cells
- How to calculate cell potential using reduction potentials
- How to balance redox reactions using half-reactions
- Oxidation numbers
- Common oxidizing and reducing agents
- How to convert between EMF, Gibbs' free energy, and equilibrium constant

GENERAL CHEMISTRY PRACTICE SET

Answer Key

Passage I (Questions 1–5)
1. A
2. B
3. A
4. A
5. A

Passage II (Questions 6–10)
6. C
7. C
8. A
9. C
10. B

Passage III (Questions 11–15)
11. D
12. B
13. C
14. D
15. A

Passage IV (Questions 16–20)
16. B
17. C
18. A
19. C
20. A

Passage V (Questions 21–25)
21. D
22. D
23. D
24. B
25. A

Passage VI (Questions 26–30)
26. A
27. C
28. A
29. D
30. D

Passage VII (Questions 31–35)
31. A
32. A
33. C
34. D
35. B

Discrete Questions (Questions 36–45)
36. C
37. D
38. B
39. D
40. B
41. B
42. D
43. C
44. A
45. A

GENERAL CHEMISTRY PRACTICE SET

Answers and Explanations

Passage I (Questions 1–5)

1. A

This question requires you to recall and apply the formula for formal charge on an atom. The formal charge on an atom is given by the following equation:

Formal charge = valence electrons in neutral atom – non-bonding electrons – 1/2 bonding electrons

Neutral hydrogen has one valence electron. A hydrogen atom in polywater has no nonbonding electrons and four bonding electrons. Therefore, the formal charge on a given H atom in polywater is: $1 - 0 - 2 = -1$, answer choice **A**. Usually hydrogen would have a formal charge of zero since it would only be involved in one bond, but in this case we see a negative formal charge for hydrogen because it is involved in more than one bond.

2. B

In this question, you're going to need to combine your critical reading skills with your knowledge of general chemistry. The passage describes a very intricate mechanism for producing polywater and does not support the fact that polywater can be produced in a variety of conditions, so choice **B** is ideal.

Choice A is incorrect because polywater has a higher index of refraction than normal water and so would bend light more towards the normal (recall from Snell's Law that the angle of refraction will be smaller than the angle of incidence).

$$n_1 \sin\theta_1 = n_2 \sin\theta_2$$

So, if $n_{poly} > n_{water}$ then $\theta_{poly} < \theta_{water}$. Choice **C** is incorrect because polywater is 40% more dense than water. So, an equal mass of polywater will have a smaller volume. Choice **D** is incorrect because the passage states that polywater has a freezing-point of –40°C.

3. A

Focus on Hypothesis 2. We already know that vapor pressure and boiling point are colligative properties that depend on the number of particles in a solution, so assuming that Hypothesis 2 is correct and that polywater is merely an aqueous solution with dissolved materials, its vapor pressure would be lower than that of normal water, and its boiling point would be higher.

4. A

Many MCAT students choose the wrong answer not because they don't know the science, but because they end up getting bogged down by algebra. This is one example of a time when a question hinges not only on our conceptual understanding, but on our ability to perform algebraic operations fastidiously. Because the temperature is kept constant during the expansion process, we may use Boyle's Law to find the final pressure in the chamber. Boyle's Law states that $P_iV_i = P_fV_f$. Now, simply solve for $P_f = \dfrac{P_iV_i}{V_f}$.

Answer choice **C** might seem tempting as it uses the ideal gas law form, solved for pressure, but the question stem asks for the final pressure, and the volume in **C** is an initial volume.

5. A

In this question, we must take care to consider the ramifications of each answer choice in relation to both hypotheses if we are to distinguish the individual validity of each. If the mass of the capillary remained unchanged (answer choice **A**), this would weaken Hypothesis 2, which states that the contaminants in polywater dissolved from the quartz capillary. Weakening Hypothesis 2 would support Hypothesis 1.

Choice **B** is incorrect. If deionization of polywater increased its freezing temperature, this would indicate that polywater contained dissolved solids and would provide support for Hypothesis 2. Choice **C** is incorrect. If Hypothesis 2 is correct, we expect polywater to have a higher boiling point than normal water because dissolved solids increase the boiling point of solvents. Choice **D** is incorrect because the temperature of the second chamber is irrelevant as long as it is below the boiling point of water—keeping it at 50°C and seeing similar results would neither support nor weaken Hypothesis 1.

Passage II (Questions 6–10)

6. C

This question basically requires you to consult the phase diagram at the given values for temperature and pressure. The phase that exists at a particular temperature and pressure is the most thermodynamically favored phase. Thus, when the solid, frozen sample is placed in the chamber, it must be the solid frozen phase that is most stable. By the same reasoning, the most thermodynamically favorable phase of water at atmospheric pressure and room temperature (25°C) is the liquid phase.

We can look at the phase diagram for pure water provided in the passage to give us a hint about the most stable phase

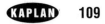

109

of dilute coffee at –20°C and 1 atm. Recall that –20°C is 273 K – 20K = 253 K. At 250 K and 1 atm, water is in the solid phase. We cannot rely solely on the information in the phase diagram because the properties of a solution (like coffee) can differ from those of a pure substance (like water), but in this case, the division between solid and the other two phases is far enough from the point we're examining that we can qualitatively predict the solid phase for dilute coffee and arrive at answer choice **C**.

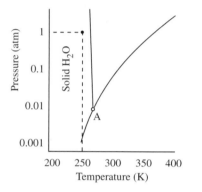

Choice **D** is incorrect. Plasma is sometimes considered the fourth phase of matter. It is a very high temperature, ionized gas that behaves like a gas in many ways but has additional properties, like conduction of electricity, which differentiate it from the gas phase.

7. C

What is the best approach to this question? Focus on the fact that the question stem says "could be." In other words, you don't have to do calculations, just recognize that the values given in the answer choices are going to fall into a few different categories, and choose the pair of values that best fits the information you gleaned from the passage. The passage describes the brewing of coffee and indicates that some amount of solid, 2.11 g, is dissolved or suspended in a 0.48-L sample of the beverage. The boiling point and freezing point of a liquid are colligative properties. That is, they are affected by the concentration of dissolved solutes in the solution. The boiling point of a liquid is raised by the presence of solutes (boiling point elevation) while the freezing point is decreased (freezing point depression). Therefore, while we do not have sufficient information to calculate the numerical values, we can predict, qualitatively, that coffee will have a higher boiling point and a lower freezing point than does pure water. The question stem states that 0°C is equivalent to 273 K. Therefore, we expect coffee to have a boiling point higher than 373 K (100°C) and lower than 273 K (0°C). Only choice **C** has the expected values.

8. A

Before answering the question, it is important to consider what factors can affect reaction rates. Temperature, concentration of reactants, catalysts, and the medium in which the reaction takes place can all have an effect on the rate of the reaction.

The question stem discusses the factors that make freeze drying a better means of producing dehydrated coffee. It is up to us to determine why freeze drying promotes these factors:

1. The oxidation rate is lower (due to low partial pressure of oxygen in the vacuum chamber)
2. The rate of protein denaturation is lower (due to lower temperatures)
3. There is reduced transport of volatile soluble flavor and aroma species (because the coffee is frozen solid)

Any changes that improve these properties would tend to produce a higher quality coffee. Filling the chamber with helium gas reduces the rate of oxidation in the coffee by decreasing (to zero) the partial pressure of oxygen in the chamber (answer choice **A**).

Choice **B** is incorrect because raising the final temperature from –5°C to 0°C would tend to increase the reaction rates, including the rate of oxidation, thereby lowering the coffee quality. Choice **C** is incorrect because increasing the surface area between the oxygen in the chamber and the frozen coffee would increase the oxidation reaction rate. This is similar to providing a larger catalytic surface on which the reaction (oxidation) can take place. Choice **D** is incorrect because compressing the sample of frozen coffee with a piston would not have a significant effect on the important reaction rates. Recall that solids are generally incompressible. While this may increase the pressure on the frozen coffee, it doesn't affect the concentration of oxygen, the flow of materials in the coffee, or the rate of protein denaturation. In an extreme case, it is possible that the increased pressure on the frozen coffee would cause it to melt. You can see in the phase diagram that increased pressure (be it pressure applied by the atmosphere or by a piston) can cause water to undergo a phase change from solid to liquid.

9. C

Heat transfer is the transfer of thermal energy from a hot body to a cooler one. Radiation is the transfer of heat by electromagnetic (infrared) waves. This kind of heat transfer can occur even through a vacuum and is the means by which heat flows from the sun to the earth. Conduction is the transfer of heat between two physically touching bodies. Convection is the transport of heat by the movement of a fluid, like steam or liquid nitrogen. For example, a radiator radiates heat into a room, but the heat is transferred to the metal radiator by the flow of steam through its pipes (convection).

In Experiment 2, heat flows from the sample by radiation to the chamber walls, conduction from the metal wall to the pipes containing the liquid nitrogen, then convection by the movement of the liquid nitrogen away from the chamber (answer **C**).

Note that in Experiment 1, the heat flows in the opposite direction. The steam carries the heat to the chamber by convection, the heat is transferred from the pipes to the chamber walls by conduction and then radiated to the sample.

What if the sample were in direct contact with the chamber walls? In this case, heat would be conducted from the sample to the walls, then conducted from the walls to the pipes, then carried away by convection. However, conduction then convection is not an option among the answer choices and choice **C** is the only possibility.

10. B
Since the question stem finishes by asking about the temperature of the water *over time*, we should approach it by considering each element of the process separately in order to come up with a plot. The question states that first the pressure is reduced to 0.05 atm. This is our cue not to confuse the plot at 1 atm with that at 0.05 atm when we start examining the answer choices. During this time, the temperature will decrease since pressure is decreasing and volume remains constant. (The size of the chamber hasn't been altered.) So let's consider the phase diagram of water at 0.05 atm:

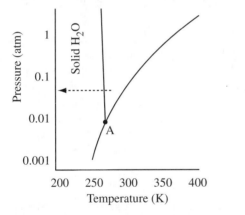

As heat is extracted, the water will cool to its freezing point at 0.05 atm. At the freezing point it will begin to freeze. Once all the water has frozen, the ice will begin to cool below its freezing point as more heat is extracted. From the phase diagram we can see that the freezing point of water at 0.05 atm is a little higher than the freezing point at 1 atm. This is because water, unlike most liquids, expands as it freezes.

Freezing is an exothermic process and the heat released is extracted by the heat sink at a constant rate. All of the heat that is extracted during the freezing process comes from the $\Delta H_{freezing}$ and the temperature of the H_2O remains constant

until it is completely frozen. This is the part of the plot where the line is essentially horizontal. At this point, the temperature of the ice begins to fall from the freezing point.

In the graph, we expect to see a downward slope until the freezing point is reached. We expect a horizontal plateau of temperature, or isotherm, as the water freezes, then another downward slope as the ice cools.

Only choices **A** and **B** have this kind of profile. Choice **A** represents the temperature profile for water at 1 atm, while choice **B** is correct for the given pressure of 0.05 atm.

Choices **C** and **D** can be ruled out because they indicate instantaneous changes in temperature (the vertical portions of the plot.) Temperature changes can occur rapidly, but not instantaneously because heat flow cannot be infinite, so vertical lines in a temperature vs. time plot will never be observed.

Passage III (Questions 11–15)

11. D
This is one of those times when we just have to commit certain pieces of information to memory. The colors of visible light, in the order of increasing energy and frequency, are ROYGBIV: red, orange, yellow, green, blue, indigo, violet. The way we can remember that red is on the low-frequency, low-energy end and that violet is on the high-frequency, high-energy end is to recall the types of radiation adjacent to visible light in the electromagnetic spectrum: infra*red* and ultra*violet*.

12. B
The best strategy here is to count the number of sp^2-hybridized carbon atoms in the 3-aminophthalate anion and in the luminol molecule. There are 8 carbon atoms in luminol: the six that form the benzene ring, and the two carbonyl carbons. They all form a double bond and two single bonds and are hence sp^2-hybridized. In the 3-aminophthalate anion, none of the carbon atoms was removed and all of the atoms remain sp^2-hybridized; the only difference is that the amide functionalities have been converted into carboxylates. The two carbon atoms, however, are still carbonyl carbons, so the number of sp^2-hybridized carbon atoms remains unchanged.

13. C
The first thing to recognize when considering the question stem here is the phrase *not all of the energy*, indicating that most of the excited state energy is emitted during luminescence, but that some is dissipated through the collisions. From this we can assume that whatever phenomenon we observe will exhibit a bit of blurriness. The amount of energy dissipated through collisions will

obviously depend on such factors as the number of collisions and their efficiencies. Hence, the energy that will ultimately be radiated is indeterminate: It can be as high as the difference in energy between A* and A, but more likely it is less than this amount because part of the difference is dissipated through collisions. We know that the energy of a photon is related to its frequency by E = hf, where E is the energy, h is Planck's constant, and f is the frequency. The photon emitted during chemiluminescence carries with it the excess energy that the chemical species possesses. In other words, the energy carried by the photon is, in the simplest case, the difference in energy between A* and A, where A stands for some generic chemical species that is formed in the reaction producing the luminescence. In short, a range of energy values can be carried by the photons, resulting in a range of frequencies (and hence wavelengths). Therefore, choice **C** is correct.

Choice **A** is incorrect. If the total pressure were increased, the frequency of collisions would also increase. More energy would then be dissipated via collisions than by luminescence. Choice **B** is also incorrect because the exact reverse should be the result of collisional deactivation. As described above, a higher pressure would increase the probability that energy is dissipated by collisions rather than radiated in the form of luminescence. In fact, gas-phase chemiluminescent reactions are often carried out under conditions of low total pressure to enhance the intensity. (One may argue that if the pressure were increased by increasing the concentration of the gas-phase reactants, this would increase the rate of reaction and hence the intensity. This, however, would not be a direct effect of collisional deactivation, which is what we are asked for.) Choice **D** is incorrect because when the energy is dissipated through collisions, the species moves towards the ground state. It may not luminesce (if all of its energy is dissipated through collisions), but it will not remain in the excited state.

14. D

The key to quickly answering this question is to recognize that three of the four choices have eleven electrons in their Lewis dot structures, while the fourth has only ten. Even without knowing anything about the compound, the fact that one is drastically different from the others means that it will probably be the answer to the question. Still, let's consider exactly what is going on in this question: Nitrogen has five valence electrons while oxygen has six. NO thus has a total of 11 valence electrons. The structure shown in choice D has only 10 valence electrons: 3 pairs of bonding electrons gives 6 electrons, plus two lone pairs which provides another 4 electrons. It does not have the correct number of electrons and thus cannot be a correct Lewis

structure. All the other structures have 11 valence electrons.

15. A

This is a complicated and involved question, so the best approach is to map out exactly what is being asked, compare that with what we know from the passage, and go from there. The answer choices have two parts each: the order in which Fe^{2+} ions encounter the organic species and are introduced into the luminol-peroxide mixture, and the concentration of the organic species relative to the concentration of Fe^{2+}. So, the thing to do here is to sketch out which combination of conditions will produce the results we want, then match this to our answer choices. In order for the intensity to be suppressed, the Fe^{2+} ions must be complexed with the organic species whose concentration we are trying to determine. This complexing must occur before the Fe^{2+} can react with the luminol-peroxidase solution; otherwise luminescence will be generated at its full intensity before there is a chance for the complexing to occur. Furthermore, the concentration of Fe^{2+} must be higher than that of the organic species. If this were not the case, we would not observe any luminescent signal at all, and we would not get any quantitative information about the concentration of the organic species, other than the fact that it is greater than that of Fe^{2+}.

Passage IV (Questions 16–20)

16. B

The question stem asks for the approximate mass percent of chloride ion in the original sample, so we should proceed to calculate it using any approximations necessary to lighten the workload. As with the majority of MCAT questions, the answer choices provided are far enough apart in magnitude that we can make reasonable approximations and still arrive at the correct answer. The mass percent of chloride ions is defined as:

$$\frac{\text{mass of chloride ions}}{\text{mass of sample}} \times 100\%$$

The passage states that the unknown sample had a mass of 0.2020 g. We need to calculate the mass of the chloride ions. The mass of AgCl formed was 0.3485 g, and for each mole AgCl formed, one mole of chloride ions was present in the original sample. The dimensional setup for the stoichiometry is as follows:

$$0.3485\text{g AgCl} \times \frac{1 \text{ mol AgCl}}{(107.9 + 35.5)\text{g AgCl}}$$

$$\times \frac{1 \text{ mol Cl}^-}{1 \text{ mol AgCl}} \times \frac{35.5 \text{ g Cl}^-}{1 \text{ mol Cl}^-}$$

After canceling units and approximating, we obtain:

$$(0.35 \times \frac{1}{140} \times 35\text{g})\text{Cl}^- = \frac{0.35}{4} \text{ g Cl}^- = 0.09 \text{ g Cl}^-$$

The percent by mass is therefore approximately:

$$\frac{0.09 \text{ g Cl}}{0.20 \text{ g sample}} \times 100\%$$

which is a bit less than 50%. Choice **B** is therefore the correct answer.

17. C

Since the question stem asks which of the choices would have the least effect on the accuracy of the results, we should examine the consequences of each answer choice before making our selection. The gist of the procedure is that chloride ion is precipitated, as AgCl, by reaction with excess silver ion. The precipitate is then washed to remove unreacted silver ion, and filtered and dried quickly enough to avoid unwanted side reactions. Choice **C** is correct because the presence of sodium ions, and additional nitrate ions, will not result in the formation of any additional product. Nor will they prevent precipitation of AgCl in any way. Nitrate is a spectator ion in the procedure described; sodium would be another spectator ion if it were present.

Choice **A** can be eliminated because, according to Reaction 2, exposure to light will cause the reduction of silver ions to metallic silver with the concurrent release of chlorine gas. This reaction, if it occurs appreciably, will result in a decrease in the mass of AgCl recovered and, consequently, an artificially low chloride determination. Answer choice **B** can be eliminated because K_{sp}, as an equilibrium constant, will be affected by a change in temperature. Since the calculations are, at least partially, based on the assumption that precipitation is nearly complete, any increase in the temperature will put this assumption in doubt, and therefore affect the accuracy of the analysis. Recall that an increase in temperature usually leads to an increase in solubility. Choice **D** can be eliminated, since hydrochloric acid, which is dissociated into H^+ and Cl^- will react with any remaining silver ions on the surface of the precipitate to form additional AgCl.

18. A

Since we're asked about precipitation in the question stem, we know our calculations will involve dilution, the common ion effect, and K_{sp} calculations as well as a general understanding of the meaning of K_{sp}. Chloride ions precipitate out to form solid AgCl upon encountering the silver ions from the silver nitrate ($AgNO_3$). Precipitation will occur if the ion product, $[Ag^+][Cl^-]$ is greater than K_{sp}. Hence, the concentration of chloride ions in solution (unprecipitated) is also dependent on the concentration of silver ions present (as well as on the solubility of AgCl). The concentration of the silver nitrate solution, before it is added to the sample to be analyzed, is 0.2 M. From the stoichiometry of the compound, we see that there is a 1:1 ratio between $AgNO_3$ and Ag^+, and so the concentration of

silver ions is also originally 0.2 M. This is, however, diluted as it is added to the 100 mL of the other solution, giving a final volume of about 120 mL. The new concentration is calculated as:

$$M_1V_1 = M_2V_2$$

$$(0.2\ M)(20 \text{ mL}) = M_2(120 \text{ mL})$$

$$M_2 = 4/120\ M = 1/30\ M\ Ag^+$$

The necessary concentration of Cl^- can then be determined from the silver ion concentration and the K_{sp} of AgCl:

$$K_{sp} = [Ag^+][Cl^-] =>$$

$$[Cl^-] = K_{sp}/[Ag^+] = 1.56 \times 10^{-10}/(1/30), \text{ or}$$

$$[Cl^-] = 1.5 \times 10^{-10} \times 30 = 4.5 \times 10^{-9}\ M$$

Note that it is not necessary to carry out this last multiplication, as only choice **A** is larger than 1.56×10^{-10}.

19. C

In this question, we're going to use our analysis of the passage in tandem with our general knowledge of common substances. We know that the precipitate described in the passage was white, so the precipitate obtained in the other experiment must be contaminated with something else. Choice **A** is incorrect since nitrate ions, like those in the silver nitrate solution, are colorless; we know this because the nitric acid solution was colorless. Choice **B** is incorrect because, as described in an earlier question, elevated temperatures would decrease the yield of AgCl but would not affect its color. In fact, since crystallization is slower at higher temperatures, it would be less likely that extra silver ions become trapped in the crystal lattice as it forms. Choice **D** is incorrect because the passage specifically describes the formation of a "fine, white" silver chloride precipitate. Therefore, Choice **C** is correct; since silver metal has a gray color, when it is mixed in with a white precipitate, the resulting solid will have a faint violet color.

20. A

The key to answering this question quickly and correctly is recognizing that in the passage, we learned that a wet silver chloride precipitate is susceptible to photodecomposition. Therefore, if the silver chloride solution must be stored overnight before filtration, we must guard against the photodecomposition side reaction by protecting the sample from light. Therefore, choice **A** is correct. Choice **B** is incorrect because the passage tells us that the silver chloride precipitate formed immediately, so extra time will not result in a higher mass of precipitate. Choice **C** is incorrect because solvent evaporation does not affect the mass of recovered precipitate—the precipitate would be left behind if the solvent were to evaporate. Choice **D** is incorrect because exposure to chlorine vapors could only

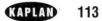

increase the mass of the precipitate using stray silver ions in solution, resulting in a higher (not lower) result.

Passage V (Questions 21–25)

21. D

The question stem asks about the inversion temperature of various gases. Since the inversion temperature is given in the passage as $2a/Rb$, a high inversion temperature results from a large a and/or a small b. With questions of this type, it is important to know how to make prudent approximations. We will try to come up with estimates of the quantity a/b for each gas, but note first of all that helium can be easily eliminated since its a and b are of the same magnitude, whereas for the other gases a is bigger than b by a factor of 10 or more.

$$H_2: \frac{0.244}{0.0266} = \sim 10$$

$$N_2: \frac{1.39}{0.0391} = \sim \frac{1.4}{0.04} = \sim \frac{140}{4} = 35$$

$$(>10; \text{ eliminate choice } \mathbf{B})$$

$$CH_4: \frac{2.25}{0.0428} = \sim \frac{2.25}{0.04} \; (> \frac{1.4}{0.04}, \text{ which is the value for } N_2)$$

Hence CH_4 has the highest a/b value, and should thus be expected to have the highest inversion temperature.

22. D

The magnitude of work associated with the volume change of a gas at constant pressure is given by $|W| = |P\Delta V|$, where P is the pressure and ΔV is the change in volume. If the gas expands, it does work on the environment, whereas if it contracts, work is done on the gas. If net work is done, then the magnitude of the work done by the gas upon expansion must be greater than the magnitude of the work done on the gas in contraction. Let us apply this to the Joule-Thomson experiment.

Let us focus our attention on the particular amount of gas that is transferred from chamber 1 to chamber 2. This gas is compressed against pressure P_1. The change in volume associated with this compression is its entire volume, since all of it is removed from chamber 1. In other words, its volume change upon compression is the volume change of chamber 1 as a whole, i.e. ΔV_1. The amount of work done on the transferred gas therefore has a magnitude of $|P_1\Delta V_1|$.

This gas enters chamber 2 where it expands against a pressure P_2. The volume change of this expansion is the volume change of chamber 2 as a whole, i.e. ΔV_2. So the gas does work of magnitude $|P_2\Delta V_2|$. As mentioned at the beginning, if net work is done, then $|W|_{\text{expansion}} > |W|_{\text{compression}}$. Hence $|P_2\Delta V_2| > |P_1\Delta V_1|$.

23. D

Although it may be tempting to answer this question using the Ideal Gas Law, this is in fact a qualitative question on the behavior of real gases. When an ideal gas is compressed to half its initial volume at constant temperature, we know from Boyle's law (or the ideal gas law) that its pressure doubles. When a real gas is compressed, however, there are two competing factors that come into play. The attractive forces become stronger as the average distance between the gas molecules decreases. This has the effect of lowering the pressure from the expected doubling. At the same time, however, the excluded volume taken up by the gas particles now constitutes a more significant fraction of the total volume. The effective volume available to the gas molecules, therefore, is less than half of the initial effective volume. The pressure is therefore expected to be more than doubled from this factor. Which factor dominates depends on the actual numerical values of such parameters as a, b, initial pressure, etc.

24. B

When answering this question, it's worthwhile to notice that we don't need to have read the passage to answer correctly. We have three options. The first is to recall what the plot looks like from our chemistry studies. The second option is to think through the behavior of real gases in order to generate our own plot and compare it with the answer choices. Our third option is to examine the repercussions of each answer choice and decide which is the best. This backsolving approach is going to be quickest if we can't immediately remember how the plot should look. When the separation between two neutral particles is relatively large, there is a weak attractive force between them because of van der Waals forces. These forces tend to draw the particles closer together, and hence the potential energy is lowered as the two approach each other from far away. This by itself is sufficient to enable us to pick **B** as the correct answer. For completeness, let us continue with the analysis. The lowering of the potential energy does not continue indefinitely as eventually the particles get so close together that their electron clouds start to repel. Beyond a certain point, then, the potential energy starts to increase as the separation keeps decreasing. This is illustrated in the curve shown in choice **B**.

25. A

This is another one of those questions that follow a passage but don't really require you to have read the passage to answer correctly. We're told that we have two vessels, one with argon, one with neon. If the same amount of heat is added to both samples of gases and no volume change occurs (hence W = 0), then all the heat is used to increase the internal energies of the gases. For ideal gases, the internal energy, U, is proportional to the temperature.

Since the two gases have the same initial temperature and experience the same amount of kinetic energy increase (same temperature change), they will also have the same final temperature. Choices **C** and **D** can thus be eliminated. To decide between choices **A** and **B**, we need to recognize that neon and argon have different atomic masses. Since kinetic energy is $\frac{1}{2}mv^2$, and the two have the same average kinetic energy, the less massive of the two gases will be moving more quickly. Neon is lighter than argon, which is enough for us to conclude that choice **A** must be correct.

Passage VI (Questions 26–30)

26. A
The key to answering this question correctly is recognizing which part of the passage is relevant. The energy profile, reaction mechanisms and rates-concentrations table might throw us off, so we need to stay focused on the K values given in the reaction scheme in Figure 1. K represents the ratio of products to reactants at equilibrium, so the reaction with the largest K value will proceed the furthest toward completion at equilibrium. The equilibrium constants for the three reactions are given in Figure 1. Reaction I with a $K = 3 \times 10^4$, will have proceeded the furthest toward completion once equilibrium has been established. Answer choice **A** is correct.

27. C
For this question begin by noting that the generic rate expression for this process is

$$\text{Rate} = k[tert\text{-butyl bromide}]^x[\text{OH}^-]^y$$

Then use the experimental data given in Table 1 to determine the values of x and y. First examine the changes observed between experiments 1 and 2. The concentration of hydroxide was doubled, but the initial rate remained unchanged. Therefore, rate does not depend on hydroxide concentration, so $y = 0$. Now focus on experiments 1 and 3. When the concentration of tert-butyl bromide is doubled, the initial rate also doubles, so $x = 1$. Therefore, the rate expression is

$$\text{Rate} = k[tert\text{-butyl bromide}].$$

28. A
Although the question specifically refers to Reaction I, it is really asking us to consider the consequences of running any reaction at a higher temperature. Rate constants and equilibrium constants are both affected by temperature. Let's consider how. The temperature dependence of the rate constant is explained by the Arrhenius equation:

$$\ln k = \ln A - \frac{E_a}{RT}$$

In order for a collision between two species to result in a chemical reaction, the two species must have sufficient kinetic energy to overcome the activation energy barrier for that reaction. As temperature increases, so does kinetic energy. With a higher proportion of molecules having a kinetic energy greater than the activation energy for a reaction, more collisions will result in a reaction and the rate will increase. Therefore, the important thing to recognize is that as the temperature increases, so does the rate constant. You can now eliminate answer choices **B** and **D**. Now let's consider the equilibrium constant. The temperature dependence of the equilibrium constant is described by the equation $\Delta G = -RT \ln K$, where ΔG is the standard free energy change of the reaction. If we solve for $\ln K$, we find an inverse relationship between K and temperature. This means that as temperature changes, so will the rate constant. Since both the equilibrium and the rate constant change with temperature, the correct answer choice is **A**.

29. D
Whenever a question asks about shifting an equilibrium, we should immediately think of Le Chatelier's principle. Le Chatelier's principle states if a system is subjected to a stress, it will adjust itself in order to alleviate that stress. One of the stresses a system can experience relates to the concentrations of reactants and products. For Reaction II, the alkene will be favored if bromide can be removed from the reactant side of the equilibrium. This could be accomplished by precipitating the bromide ion through addition of silver nitrate.

30. D
In order to answer this question correctly, we must consider the functions of a catalyst. Adding a catalyst causes the rate of the forward reaction to increase because the activation energy for the forward process with a catalyst is lower than the activation energy without the catalyst. We know this from the Boltzmann distribution. However, the activation energy for the reverse reaction is also lowered by addition of a catalyst, so the equilibrium constant will remain the same. Addition of a catalyst affects the forward and reverse reactions equally, so none of the equilibrium constants will change.

Passage VII (Questions 31–35)

31. A
Although the last phrase in the question stem does not explicitly say "standard reduction half-reactions" but rather "standard half-reaction," the question does state that E values are for reduction half-reactions. You must be aware of this in order to master this type of question. This means that from left to right, we have "oxidized form,

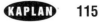

reduced form" as the half reaction to which E refers. A metal such as gold, which according to the passage does not corrode under normal circumstances, is resistant to oxidation. You should therefore predict that a reduction reaction like $Au^+(aq) + e^- \rightarrow Au(s)$ would have a positive E relative to the hydrogen reference electrode, since the passage told us that Au is not easily corroded. At the opposite end of the spectrum, metals like Mg, as well as Group IA and IIA metals in general, are easily corroded—*oxidized*—meaning that they should have a negative E relative to hydrogen so that a spontaneous cell reaction can occur in solution. Choice **A** is correct.

32. A
Based on the wording of the question stem, we already know that we need to compare the pH with the pOH to determine why one changes and the other does not. As Table 1 shows, in strongly basic solution $[OH^-]$ remains constant with increasing temperature because the extreme pH comes from having such a large number of basic ions present—in this case, 0.032 M base. This number is much, much greater than the amount of OH^- (or H_3O^+) that comes from water—only 10^{-7} M at 25°C. The change in pK_w values from 0 to 30 yields a change in $[OH^-]$ or $[H_3O^+]$ contributed from water of less than a factor of ten, so we can see how little the temperature will affect the make-up of strongly basic or acidic solutions through changes in water self-ionization. Choice **B** is misleading in that it does contain a kernel of truth: At higher temperatures, reactants have more energy and reaction rates can go faster, and the excess base will by Le Chatelier's principle shift the position of the water equilibrium. But the excess $[OH^-]$ will not change the value of K_w—only the change in temperature does that. Choice **C**, though a true statement, does not correctly explain the behavior described in the question. That is, it does explain why the pH changes; however, it does not explain why pOH remains essentially fixed. Finally, choice **D** begins with a true statement, but then makes a false statement. Yes, pH does measure $[H^+]$. However, $[H^+]$ and $[OH^-]$ are interrelated by the autoionization of water. The point of the question is that although they *are* interrelated, the magnitude of the concentration overwhelms this relation.

33. C
To answer this question, let's first remember that reduction takes place at the cathode (mnemonic: RED CAT), while oxidation takes place at the anode (mnemonic: AN OX). Then let's focus on the crucial fact that solid metal is being dissolved (not formed), so the metal half-reaction will need to go from the neutral atom state to the ionized state. This leads us to choice **C**. Choice **A** is wrong because it shows an oxidation followed by a reduction. The question stem, however, asks for reduction followed by an oxidation

(look back: cathode first, anode second). Choice **B** is reduction and then oxidation, which could be cathodic and anodic reactions, but not for corrosion: Fe(s) in this choice is being formed, not dissolved. Finally, choice **D** is incorrect since there is no redox potential to drive this reaction.

34. D
This type of question cannot be answered by prediction—we must go through the answer choices and evaluate each one. The passage clearly states that choice **A** is true—hydronium and hydroxide ions in water determine the corrosiveness of a solution. Table 1 indicates that choice **B** is true as well. The pH changes with temperature because of the change in water's contribution to the proton concentration. However, the high concentration is unaffected by the small contribution from water. The first phrase in choice **C** was stated in the passage, and the second choice is really saying the same thing as the first—temperature is representative of kinetic energies of solution particles, and more kinetic energy means a greater chance of reaction, or in this case corrosion. So from process of elimination this leaves choice **D** as the answer. Table 1 indicates that pH decreases with increasing temperature—therefore corrosivity decreases.

35. B
This question challenges us to draw conclusions from what we read in the passage and observed in Table 1, using our knowledge of acid-base equilibria and pH trends. This is an ideal time to *predict* the answer before reading all the answer choices. If in strongly basic solutions the pOH stays fixed, then in strongly acidic solutions the pH should stay fixed. The pK_w will do exactly the same thing whether you are in acid or base solution, so Table 1 shows that it will decrease (more products at equilibrium) at higher temperature. Likewise, water will produce more OH^- ions at higher temperature and so the pOH will decrease to show this behavior, just as the pH decreased in highly basic solutions. Remember that in both cases—strong acid or base—the water autoionization reaction is producing more H^+ and more OH^- with increasing temperature. We only see a change in the amount of the more dilute component. Choice **B** reflects these predictions.

36. C
The first step in solving a percentage yield question is to determine the limiting reagent. The balanced chemical equation shows H_2S reacting with SO_2 in a 2:1 molar ratio. 204 kg of H_2S corresponds to:

$$\frac{204 \times 10^3 \text{ g}}{(2 \times 1.0 + 32.0)\text{g/mol}} = 6 \times 10^3 \text{ mol } H_2S$$

256 kg of SO_2 corresponds to:

$$\frac{256 \times 10^3 \text{ g}}{(32.0 + 2 \times 16.0) \text{ g/mol}} = 4 \times 10^3 \text{ mol } SO_2$$

The molar ratio of H_2S to SO_2 is $6 \times 10^3 : 4 \times 10^3 = 6:4 = 1.5:1$. Since there are only 1.5 moles of H_2S for every mole of SO_2 (instead of 2:1), H_2S is the limiting reagent.

The chemical equation shows that the Claus process produces 3 moles of S_2 for every 2 moles of H_2S. Hence, if we start with 6×10^3 mol of H_2S, the theoretical yield of the reaction would be:

$$\text{theoretical yield} = \frac{3 \text{ moles S}}{2 \text{ moles } H_2S} \times (6 \times 10^3 \text{ moles } H_2S)$$

$$= 9 \times 10^3 \text{ moles S}$$

However, the question stem tells us that we only end up with 224 kg of S. This corresponds to 7×10^3 moles S:

$$\text{actual yield} = \frac{224 \times 10^3 \text{ g S}}{32 \text{ g/mol S}} = 7 \times 10^3 \text{ moles S}$$

Therefore the percentage yield of sulfur is:

$$\text{percentage yield} = \frac{\text{actual yield}}{\text{theoretical yield}} \times 100\%$$

$$= \frac{7 \times 10^3 \text{ moles S}}{9 \times 10^3 \text{ moles S}} \times 100\% = 77\%, \text{ choice } \mathbf{C}.$$

37. D
An equilibrium constant of 0.05 means that at equilibrium the ratio of product $[A^-][H_3O^+]$ to the amount $[HA]$ is 5:100. This eliminates choices **A** and **B**. If we forget that there are *two* products in the formula for K,

$$K = \frac{[H_3O^+][A^-]}{[HA]}, \text{ not } K = \frac{[A-]}{[HA]}$$

then choice **C** would appear to be correct. With an equilibrium constant $K \ll 1$, the reactant HA undergoes little ionization (also called hydrolysis or dissociation) in water. Choice **D** is therefore the correct answer. Choice **A** could appear to be correct if we were looking at the balanced equation (a 1:1 mole ratio) and ignoring the value of K. Balanced equations tell us only how many individual product species will be present at equilibrium relative to one reactant species, not how many of those reactants are actually converted to products by the time the equilibrium is established.

38. B
A Lewis base is a compound that can donate an electron pair. Choice **A**, chlorous acid, will not act as a Lewis base. Rather, it is an Arrhenius acid, capable of donating a hydrogen ion in solution. Choice **B**, hydrazine, consists of two nitrogens bonded to each other and to two hydrogen atoms each. A nitrogen atom has a valence of five, and when it's bonded to another nitrogen and two hydrogens, it's only using three of its five valence electrons. Therefore, each nitrogen will have a pair of unbonded electrons. This makes hydrazine able to act as an electron-pair donor, or

Lewis base, so choice **B** is the correct answer. Looking at the other choices, choice **C**, an ammonium ion, is not a Lewis base. In fact, it's the conjugate acid of ammonia. Choice **D** is boron trifluoride. The boron atom has three valence electrons, each of which is involved in a covalent bond with a fluorine atom, and thus has no electron pairs to donate. Once again, choice **B** is the correct answer.

39. D
Perhaps the easiest way to solve a problem such as this is to imagine a particular sample mass of the compound. We shall choose a mass of 100 grams for convenience, though any mass we use will lead us to the correct answer. Because the oxide of arsenic contains only arsenic and oxygen, a 100 gram sample would contain 65.2 grams of arsenic and the remainder, 34.8 grams, must be oxygen. To find the ratio between these two elements in the compound we divide the mass of arsenic by the atomic weight of arsenic, 74.7 grams per mole, and the mass of oxygen by the atomic weight of oxygen, 16 grams per mole. This will give the mole ratio between arsenic and oxygen in the compound. To convert to a more easily useful ratio, we divide both by the lowest number of the two, here arsenic. This gives us a ratio of 1 mole arsenic to 2.5 moles oxygen. Multiply both of these to get 2 moles arsenic per 5 moles of oxygen. This corresponds to As_2O_5, the formula in choice **D**.

40. B
This question tests your understanding of VSEPR, the Valence Shell Electron Pair Repulsion theory of molecular geometry. First, we must determine the molecular geometry of SO_2 and then compare this to the answer choices. Using Lewis dot structures, we can get an idea of the number of bonds and lone electron pairs. Use the periodic table in your test booklet to determine the number of electrons in the valence shells of different elements. Sulfur (S) has 6 electrons in its valence shell as does each oxygen (O) in its valence shell.

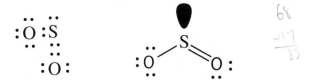

VSEPR proposes that the repulsion between electron pairs makes molecules adopt shapes that have the greatest separation between the electron pairs. The lone pair of electrons in SO_2 push the atoms into a bent configuration. Note that when we discuss molecular geometry, we are concerned with the arrangements of the bonds, not the arrangements of the electron pairs. Note also that the diagram above only shows one of the resonance structures of SO_2. In reality, the double bond is shared equally

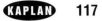

between the two NO bonds.

Now let's consider the answer choices.

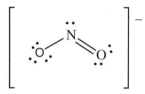

Answer choice **A**, CO_2, has a linear configuration. It has two double bonds of carbon to oxygen. CO_2 does not have a bent structure.

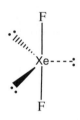

Answer choice **B** is the correct answer. NO_2^- has a bent molecular structure. Again, the diagram above only shows one of the resonance structures of NO_2^-. These bonds are bent by the influence of the lone pair of electrons. Note that this is a negative ion, which explains the extra electron. We will consider the other answer choices for completeness.

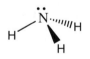

Answer choice **C**, XeF_2, has a linear molecular structure. Note that the electron pairs are arranged in a trigonal bipyramidal geometry. However, when we consider just the bonds to other nuclei, the geometry is linear.

Answer choice **D**, NH_3, has three hydrogens bonded to the central nitrogen, so we can already determine that it will not have the bent structure. The bent structure requires that there be 2 atoms bonded to a central atom. NH_3 has a trigonal pyramidal structure. The three hydrogens are pushed out of the plane by the lone pair.

41. B
This question deals with the colligative properties of solutions. The first is that the presence of a solute in a solution always raises the boiling point and lowers the freezing point, relative to the boiling and freezing points of the pure solvent. A higher concentration of solute in the solution leads to a greater boiling point elevation and

freezing point depression. Thus it is clear that choice **A** is incorrect; since Solution Y's boiling point is higher than Solution X's, its freezing point must be lower as well. The second important concept is that of vapor pressure, which is the topic of both answers **B** and **D**. A solution boils when its vapor pressure is equal to the atmospheric pressure. Since solution Y is not boiling at 100.26°C and solution X is boiling, we know the vapor pressure of solution Y must be below that of solution X. Choice **B** is therefore correct, and choice **D** incorrect. Choice **C** concerns the miscibility of solutions X and Y, i.e., the solubility of the two solutions in each other. We don't have enough information to say that this answer is correct. We are not given any information about the solubilities of solutions X and Y, so Choice **C** is irrelevant.

42. D
The standard potential of a reaction is a measure of the driving force behind the reaction. When the potential is positive, as it is in this case, the reaction will take place spontaneously.

To answer this question, we must first express the balanced equation given in terms of separate oxidation and reduction equations. Once we do this, the equations you get are, for oxidation:

$$2\ Al \rightarrow 2\ Al^{3+} + 6e^-$$

and for reduction:

$$2\ Fe^{3+} + 6e^- \rightarrow 2\ Fe$$

The oxidation state of the oxide ions does not change, and therefore these are not taken into account when determining the voltage. Next, we determine and add up the standard potentials for these half reactions. The table indicates that the standard potential for the reduction of aluminum is −1.66 volts. Since in this case the aluminum is being oxidized instead of reduced, we subtract the −1.66 volts, changing its sign from minus to plus. *We do not multiply the 1.66 by two for the two moles of aluminum in the balanced equation.*

Next, we determine the reduction potential for iron from the +3 valence to 0. This is given in the table as −0.037 V. Finally, we add together the −0.037 volts from the reduction of iron with the 1.66 volts from the oxidation of aluminum. This gives us a total of 1.62 volts for the total reaction, choice **D**.

43. C
The $\Delta H°$ for a reaction can be calculated as the difference between the heat of formation of the products and that of the reactants.

$$\Delta H°_{reaction} = \Delta H°_{f(products)} - \Delta H°_{f(reactants)}$$

Recall that heat of formation is the heat of the reaction that produces 1 mol of the material in question from pure elements in their standard states. The heat of formation of elements in their standard states is zero. The passage provides the reaction for formation of Fe_3O_4:

$$3\ Fe(s) + 2\ O_2(g) \rightarrow Fe_3O_4(s)\Delta H - 1118.4\ kJ \cdot mol^{-1}$$

So we can determine the heat of formation of Fe_2O_3 from the first equation and the $\Delta H°_f$ of Fe_3O_4 given by the equation above.

$$\Delta H°_{reaction} = 4(\Delta H°_f Fe_3O_4) + \Delta H°_f O_2 - 6(\Delta H°_f Fe_2O_3)$$
$$+472 = 4(-1118.4) + 0 - 6(\Delta H°_f Fe_2O_3)$$
$$4944 = -6(\Delta H°_f Fe_2O_3)$$
$$\Delta H°_f Fe_2O_3 = -824\ kJ \cdot mol^{-1}$$

answer choice **C**. We should, of course, use approximations judiciously to save time.

44. A
The key to answering this question correctly is remembering the definition of density. Remember that we can manipulate the equation into a more useful form and then think over what else we would need to know to answer the question. Recall that density is mass divided by volume. If we want to know the density of oxygen in a container, we need to know the mass of the oxygen divided by the volume of the oxygen. This is true regardless of the fact that there may also be other gases present in the container. Since we are required to use the formula $PV = nRT$, we'll rearrange this formula so that we have mass over volume on the left and what it is equal to, in all those other terms, on the right. First, remember that P equals pressure, V equals volume, n equals number of moles, T is temperature and R is the gas constant. How do we get mass into this equation? The number of moles of oxygen, n, is equal to the actual mass of oxygen, m, divided by the molar mass of oxygen, M. Substituting into the $PV = nRT$ equation we get $PV = m/MRT$. Next we have to rearrange the formula to solve for density, that is, mass, m, over volume, V. The final formula is $m/V = MP/RT$. Now to figure out what values to plug into the equation we need to answer two questions.

First, should we use the number of moles of oxygen in the container, or the total number of moles of gas in the container? And second, should we use the partial pressure of oxygen in the container, or the total pressure of all the gases in the container? First let's consider the number of moles. We are using the number of moles times the molecular weight of oxygen to equal the total mass of oxygen in the container. If we multiplied the molecular weight of oxygen by the total number of moles of all of the gases in the container, that would give us a value much greater than the mass of the oxygen alone. Thus we must use only the number of moles of oxygen. If we use the total pressure of all the gases, then the value on the right of our density equation could be changed by adding or subtracting other gases, even though the amount of oxygen remained constant. In order for the value on the right to be equal to the value on the left, which we just calculated based on the actual amount of oxygen present, the ratio of the pressure on the right to the number of moles of oxygen on the left must be constant. Therefore we have to use the partial pressure of oxygen together with the number of moles of oxygen, and the answer choice is **A**.

45. A
The equation needed to answer this question, which was derived by Bohr, predicts the frequency of light produced when an electron falls from one quantum level to another in a hydrogen atom, though it doesn't work for other kinds of atoms, since those have interelectronic interactions that complicate the energetics. The equation states that

$$E = -A\left(\frac{1}{n_i^2} - \frac{1}{n_f^2}\right),$$

where n_i is the first quantum number of the electron in its initial state and n_f is the first quantum number of the electron in its final state. A, which is a constant, is the amount of energy needed to remove an electron from the lowest energy level of a hydrogen atom to a point at an infinite distance away. The negative sign in front of the A is there because the electron in the question is falling *toward* the nucleus of the atom, and therefore is giving off energy. So, to get back to this question here, we have to multiply $-A$ by $1/3^2 - 1/2^2$. This comes to $-A \propto -5/36$, which is equal to 0.14 A, choice **A**.

CHAPTER SIX

Organic Chemistry

READING THE PASSAGE

Organic Chemistry Passage Types

Recall from our earlier discussion that MCAT science passages fall into one of three categories: information, experiment, and persuasive argument.

For *information* passages in Organic Chemistry, the paragraphs are often relatively short and are often accompanied by diagrams illustrating reactions or mechanisms. If the passage describes a specific laboratory technique or setup, it may contain lengthier text with a graphic of the relevant apparatuses. In chapter 5 of this section you saw an example of an Organic Chemistry information passage.

An information passage in Organic Chemistry may:

- Present a new reaction: its mechanism, its stereochemistry, factors affecting its rate, other factors.
- Present a series of related reactions, for example, different ways to synthesize a class of compounds, typical reactions that a class of compounds undergoes, etc.
- Describe the characteristics of a class of compounds
- Describe an experimental technique

Experiment passages often include a presentation of the results of one or more experiments. In Organic Chemistry, the data may be presented in a variety of forms: The percentage yield of a synthesis, a verbal summary of whether the reaction or isolation procedure is successful, a description of the appearance or spectroscopic properties of the product, etc. As a result, an experiment passage may not immediately be as easily recognizable from the visual layout of the passage. An information passage describing a synthesis, for example, would technically be categorized as an experiment passage if the reaction were framed within the context of "A student carried out the following synthesis...." In other words, identifying the passage type is not as easy for Organic Chemistry passages as it may be for the other science areas.

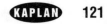

One subcategory of Organic Chemistry experiment passages, however, does merit a special mention. These are the passages detailing an extraction or purification procedure. Often the passage is accompanied by a flowchart depicting the steps; however, there may be instances when the entire procedure is only described verbally. The following is an example of such an experiment passage.

Soil contains organic matter called humus. Humus is classified into humic and nonhumic materials. Humic materials are operationally divided into three main fractions: Humic acid, fulvic acid, and humin. Because soil is heterogeneous and its composition varies from one locale to another, the actual composition of each fraction is elusive. Figure 1 shows the proposed structure for one possible component of fulvic acid.

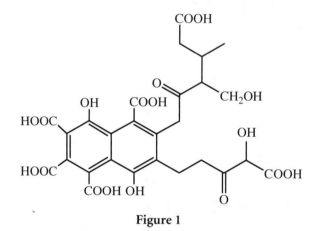

Figure 1

The traditional procedure for the separation of the three fractions from humic materials is shown in Figure 2.

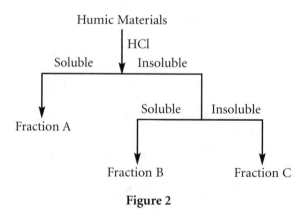

Figure 2

Some important properties of the three fractions of humic materials are listed in Table 1.

Table 1   Properties of humic materials

	Humic acid	**Fulvic acid**	**Humin**
Solubility in water	soluble in alkaline pHs	soluble at all pHs	insoluble at all pHs
Aromatic content	highly aromatic	highly aromatic	highly aromatic
Carboxylic acid content	some	high	low
Phenolic content	some	some	some
Molecular weight range (Daltons)	5,000–10,000	800–4,000	>100,000

Note that the previous passage again illustrates how the information/experiment distinction in Organic Chemistry is quite artificial at times. No actual experiment is carried out in the passage, so it could technically qualify as an information passage. However, the flowchart illustrating the separation procedure lends a very heavy experiment "flavor" to the passage.

Persuasive argument passages are relatively rare in Organic Chemistry. When they do occur, they usually appear in the form of passages presenting different proposed mechanisms for a reaction. However, it is sometimes difficult to draw the distinction between such a passage and an information passage presenting several mechanisms that are not conflicting hypotheses but are instead different mechanisms thought to operate under different conditions (acidic vs. basic, etc.). Persuasive argument passages can also resemble experiment passages in which different explanations are presented to account for a piece of data, or in which experimental data are included to support each hypothesis.

As the previous discussion suggests, categorization of passage types in Organic Chemistry is not quite as meaningful as it may be in other sciences. Nor is it especially effective in helping you answer the questions, as we shall see later. The distinction between passage types can be very fluid. In fact, regardless of what the passage deals with (and to what category it would technically belong), it will generally consist of combinations of elements, some of which are listed below:

- Diagram/chemical equation illustrating a reaction or mechanism
- Table presenting data on related compounds
- Flowchart presenting extraction series and other experimental procedures
- Prose summarizing what is already presented in a diagram
- Prose presenting new information on some aspect of the reaction(s) or on the compounds involved
- Prose detailing the experimental procedure for a reaction shown in a diagram
- Description of a proposed mechanism

Often the emphasis on one of these elements over the others is what determines the passage type.

Despite the problematic issue of categorizing Organic Chemistry passages, the technique on reading a passage still holds. You should always aim to perform two tasks on each passage: *map the passage and identify the topic.*

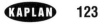

Mapping the Passage and Identifying the Topic

For Organic Chemistry passages, you need to evaluate the nature of individual blocks of text to determine what amount of attention you need to pay to the prose. Text introducing a reaction presented in a diagram often serves only to provide a context for the reaction and can be skimmed quickly for any new terms introduced; you may want to circle these terms or underline their definitions. Text detailing experimental protocol tends to be extraneous in Organic Chemistry (in contrast to Physics passages, for example). Description of a serial extraction procedure, on the other hand, merits closer attention, especially if no accompanying flowchart is included as a graphic. But again, keep in mind that you can always go back to the passage if you need to.

On the following pages, you will see the technique of mapping and identifying the topic applied to the sample passages you encountered in chapter 5 and earlier in this chapter.

> Aspirin, also known as acetylsalicylic acid, is one of the most useful and economical drugs available. It belongs to a class of drugs known as nonsteroidal anti-inflammatory drugs, and can be used to treat pain and alleviate inflammation and fever. The mechanism of aspirin's action is not fully understood, although recent research suggests that it functions by inhibiting cyclooxygenase 2, an enzyme that creates prostaglandin precursors. Prostaglandins contribute to the body's perception of pain and its inflammatory response. Prostaglandins also aid in the formation of blood clots, so aspirin thins the blood and may consequently help prevent heart disease.

Background information on aspirin. (This kind of prose, heavy on physiology and general observations, is usually not very important. Do NOT let yourself be bogged down by the details.)

> Aspirin can be synthesized from salicylic acid via the reaction shown in Figure 1.

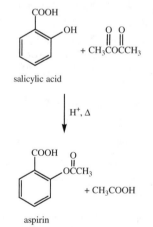

Figure 1

Reaction illustrating how aspirin can be synthesized.

> Both salicylic acid and aspirin are aromatic carboxylic acids. Carboxylic acids are generally weak acids, although they are among the strongest organic acids, with pK_a's usually in the range of 3 to 5, much lower than those of corresponding alcohols. The pK_a's of some compounds are given in Table 1.

A broadening in scope: discussion of organic acids.

Table 1   pK$_a$'s of Compounds

Compound	pK$_a$
Acetic acid	4.76
Fluoroacetic acid	2.66
Difluoroacetic acid	1.24
Trifluoroacetic acid	0.23
2,2-Dimethylpropanoic acid	5.05
Benzoic acid	4.18
p-Nitrobenzoic acid	3.43
2,4,6-Trinitrobenzoic acid	0.65
p-Methoxybenzoic acid	4.47
Phenol	9.95
Ethanol	15.9
Methanol	15.1
Water	14

Table presenting pK$_a$'s of different compounds.

Topic: The passage deals with aspirin (esp. its synthesis) and then generalizes into the topic of organic acids.

Let's map the passage we looked at before.

Soil contains organic matter called humus. Humus is classified into humic and nonhumic materials. Humic materials are operationally divided into <u>three main fractions: humic acid, fulvic acid, and humin</u>. Because soil is heterogeneous and its composition varies from one locale to another, the actual composition of each fraction is elusive. Figure 1 shows the proposed structure for one possible component of fulvic acid.

Composition of soil: some new terms introduced.

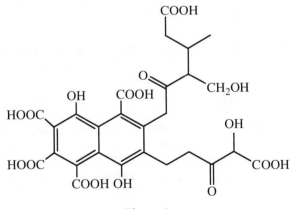

Figure 1

Structure of something that may be found in fulvic acid.

The traditional procedure for the separation of the three fractions from humic materials is shown in Figure 2.

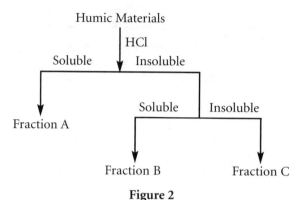

Figure 2

Some important properties of the three fractions of humic materials are listed in Table 1.

Scheme for separating the three fractions of humic materials in soil.

Table 1   Properties of humic materials

	Humic acid	**Fulvic acid**	**Humin**
Solubility in water	soluble in alkaline pHs	soluble at all pHs	insoluble at all pHs
Aromatic content	highly aromatic	highly aromatic	highly aromatic
Carboxylic acid content	some	high	low
Phenolic content	some	some	some
Molecular weight range (Daltons)	5,000–10,000	800–4,000	>100,000

Characteristics of the different fractions. Again, do NOT get bogged down with the content. At this point, a look at the categories should suffice.

Topic: The passage discusses the different components of soil and offers a scheme of separating them.

HANDLING THE QUESTIONS

For Organic Chemistry questions, wording is often straightforward and easy to grasp, which makes applying the first step of our question-answering strategy (*Understand what you are being asked*) fairly simple. This is true of most questions dealing with nomenclature, isomerism, molecular structure, etc. The following are two typical MCAT Organic Chemistry questions, together with the concepts they test:

The two organomercurial compounds in Equation 3 are:

A.   constitutional isomers.

B.   diastereomers.

C.   enantiomers.

D.   optical antipoles.

You are asked to identify the isomeric relationship between two compounds.

How many of the compounds shown in Figure 1 are aromatic?

A. 0

B. 1

C. 2

D. 3

You are asked to determine if each compound in a series satisfies the criteria for aromaticity. The question could also ask you to determine if the compounds satisfied criteria for Huckel's rule, or planarity, e.g.

A surprisingly large number of Organic Chemistry questions on the MCAT are conceptually independent of the passages they accompany. They either stand alone from the passage completely, or require only very specific data from the passage, not an in-depth understanding of it. For example, the questions may test you on outside knowledge of certain characteristics of one or more compounds mentioned in the passage.

The following question pertaining to the aspirin passage we read earlier is an example of a question that can stand alone from the passage.

Which of the following best accounts for the higher acidity of phenol compared to ethanol?

A. Phenol is hydrophobic.

B. Phenol has a higher molecular weight.

C. The benzene ring of phenol stabilizes negative charge.

D. The oxygen atom in phenol is sp^2- hybridized.

You are asked to identify the one statement from among the answer choices that explains why phenol is a stronger acid than ethanol. Nothing is needed from the passage. It is based on pure outside knowledge on acidity.

The relationship of the question to the aspirin passage is tenuous: it lies in the appearance of phenol and ethanol (and their pK_a's) in Table 1 of the passage. But the wording of the question is self-contained, and it could easily have appeared as a discrete question not accompanying any passage.

More frequently, however, you will need to go back to the passage, but only to retrieve a very specific piece of information. Consider the following questions, which could accompany the passage on soil composition.

How many stereogenic centers does the structure shown in Figure 1 contain?

A. 3

B. 6

C. 9

D. 12

Translate the question and figure out what you need to do: Identify the number of stereogenic centers (or chiral centers) contained in the molecule. (Or: Identify the number of atoms bonded to four different groups arranged in a tetrahedral geometry.)

All of the following functional groups are present in the structure shown in Figure 1 EXCEPT:

A. Alcohol

B. Carboxylic acid

C. Ester

D. Ketone

Take each answer choice and match it against the structure to see if it appears.

Translation: Need to examine Figure 1 in the passage.

For either question you need to examine the structure shown in Figure 1 (the proposed structure for a component of fulvic acid). However, for the purpose of the questions, you do not need to know what role the diagram is playing in the passage. The fact that the structure comes up during a discussion on soil composition is irrelevant to answering the question. With a slight change in wording, the structure could be included as part of the question stem and the question would be completely independent of the passage. To answer these questions you need only specific *data* from the passage.

Almost every Organic Chemistry passage on the MCAT will contain questions of this nature. Whether you need to go back to the passage or not, the important component is outside knowledge.

In Organic Chemistry, questions calling for an understanding of the passage often involve applying a reaction presented in the passage to a new set of compounds, identifying trends in data, or interpreting the result of an experiment. Success with these questions depends on critical reading of the passage and on the application of scientific reasoning in unfamiliar situations. However, even these questions usually call for outside knowledge. Consider the following question accompanying the aspirin passage:

Based on the data in Table 1, what is the expected pK_a of the following compound?

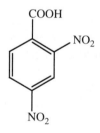

A. $pK_a < 0.65$

B. $0.65 < pK_a < 3.43$

C. $3.43 < pK_a < 4.18$

D. $pK_a > 4.18$

Determine how the structure shown is related to the ones appearing in Table 1 (using outside knowledge of nomenclature), and determine how its pK_a compares to that of other relevant compounds. Use the answer choices to decide what's demanded of you (you don't need to come up with a specific value!). Look at the relevant compounds in Table 1 to establish a trend. Use their pK_a values as benchmarks to establish the range.

 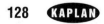

In some instances the purpose of the passage can reveal a likely line of questioning when it comes to questions calling for an understanding of the passage. For example, with a passage dealing with a multistep synthesis, you are likely to be called upon to perform one or more of the following:

- Determine what the product would be if the starting compound were a similar but distinct molecule; conversely, determine what the starting compound must have been to synthesize a similar but distinct product using the same method
- Rationalize why each step is necessary (what it accomplishes), and predict what would have been the result if the step were modified or omitted
- Predict where an isotopic label in one of the reactants ends up as a result of the reaction

An experiment passage presenting an extraction procedure, such as the passage on soil composition, may very likely be followed by questions testing your understanding of the rationale behind the scheme and the nature of the compound isolated at specific steps:

In Figure 2, Fraction B is most likely:

A. humic acid.

B. fulvic acid.

C. humin.

D. Cannot be determined from the information given.

Apply the solubility data in Figure 2 and, combining it with knowledge of the properties of the different fractions from Table 1, determine the identity of Fraction B.

This last example illustrates one point: Your evaluation of what you are being asked may undergo some refinement after you have determined exactly what in the passage is going to help you answer the question. For example, after having studied Figure 2, a more efficient characterization of your task may be: "Which of the three fractions is most likely to be insoluble in HCl but soluble in NaOH?" This, in turn, helps you narrow down what data is relevant in Table 1. As you gain experience in reading MCAT passages effectively and tackling Organic Chemistry questions, you'll learn to figure out where to find what you need and to apply your science knowledge in parallel.

A list of topics most frequently tested on the MCAT Organic Chemistry section follows. If you find you need brushing up in any of these areas, add them to your study schedule.

IN PREPARING FOR THE MCAT, I SHOULD . . .

1. Molecular Structure: Hybridization, Bonding, Polarity, Resonance, Physical Properties

- Be able to identify the hybridization of carbon atoms in different molecules
- Know the implications of hybridization on molecular geometry, bond order, etc.
- Be familiar with the characteristics of sigma versus pi bonds
- Be able to assign formal charges to atoms in a molecule
- Be able to identify polar bonds and polar molecules
- Be able to draw resonance structures and assess their stability (and hence contribution)
- Know how inductive effects and resonance stabilize charge
- Be able to identify conjugated systems, and know how conjugation affects the stability of a compound
- Know the implications of resonance on hybridization and geometry
- Be able to identify compounds capable of hydrogen bonding
- Know the trend of physical properties in hydrocarbons
- Know the common reactions of hydrocarbons, and how structural factors affect them (strain, stability of radicals, etc.)
- Be able to classify a carbon atom as methyl, primary, secondary, tertiary, or quaternary, and know the implications on reactivity
- Know how the stability of a molecule can be quantified in terms of heat of combustion, heat of hydrogenation, etc.
- Know how polarity, hydrogen bonding, molecular weight, etc., affect physical properties of compounds

2. Functional Groups

- Be able to identify the functional groups present in a molecule
- Know how to interpret condensed structural formulas
- Be aware of major characteristics of functional groups (hydrogen bonding, acidity, solubility, etc.)
- Know the fundamental rules of nomenclature for each family of compounds

3. Acidity and Basicity

- Be able to identify the most acidic proton in an organic molecule
- Know the factors affecting acidity and basicity
- Be able to account for the acidity of carboxylic acids, phenols, etc.
- Be able to predict (or rationalize) trends in acidity and basicity

4. Isomerism

- Know the definitions of the different isomers
- Be able to identify the isomeric relationship between two compounds
- Be able to identify the number of stereogenic centers in an organic molecule

 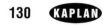

- Be able to classify a compound as chiral or achiral
- Know the origins of optical activity (specific rotation)
- Be able to identify meso compounds
- Be able to assign the absolute configuration of a chiral center
- Be able to interpret different representations of compounds: Fischer and Newman projections, etc.
- Know the conformational dynamics of ethane, butane, substituted cyclohexanes, etc.
- Know the differences/similarities in chemical and physical properties between two isomers
- Be able to identify means of separating different isomer types

5. Reactions and Syntheses: General Principles

- Be able to apply a reaction scheme given in a passage to a new set of reactants
- Be able to keep track of how bonds are formed and broken in a given mechanism by "pushing electrons," be able to apply a given, but previously unknown, mechanism to specific compounds
- Be able to visualize the mechanism in three-dimensional space to deduce the stereochemistry of the product
- Be able to deduce the structure of transition states and intermediates in a given reaction
- For a multistep synthesis, be able to recognize what happens at each step (what the step accomplishes)
- Be able to predict where an isotopic label ends up if one is employed in the reaction

6. S_N1, S_N2, E1, E2

- Know the mechanism of each reaction
- Know the rate law of each reaction
- Be able to identify reaction profiles of single-step vs. multistep reactions
- Be able to predict (in simple situations) which reaction is likely to predominate
- Be aware of the synthetic uses of the reactions
- Know the factors affecting the rate of each reaction
- Be able to predict the relative stability of carbocation intermediates
- Be able to identify good nucleophiles and good leaving groups
- Know the stereochemical implications of S_N1 versus S_N2
- Be aware of some specific examples: dehydration, solvolysis, Williamson ether synthesis, etc.
- Be able to apply Zaitsev's rule to determine the most stable elimination product

7. Addition Reactions

- Know the difference between Markovnikov and anti-Markovnikov addition;be able to predict the addition product of each
- Know the fundamental concepts of radical chemistry
- Know the mechanism of anti addition via a cyclic ion intermediate; be able to predict the product (and its most stable conformation)
- Know the stereochemistry of catalytic hydrogenation

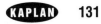

8. Aromaticity and EAS

- Be able to identify aromatic compounds by applying Huckel's rule, etc.
- Be aware of the special stability of aromatic compounds
- Be familiar with electrophilic aromatic substitution reactions: common reagents and catalysts
- Know the rate and orientation effects of different substituents; be able to classify substituents as ortho/para- or meta-directing, activating or deactivating

9. Carbonyl Chemistry

- Be able to identify different families of compounds containing the carbonyl group
- Be aware of the characteristics of the carbonyl group and how they affect its chemical reactivity
- Know the nomenclature of simple carbonyl compounds
- Know the relative position of different carbonyl compounds in the oxidation-reduction scheme
- Know the common oxidizing and reducing agents used on (or used to synthesize) carbonyl compounds
- Know the mechanism of addition reactions of aldehydes and ketones: (hemi)acetal formation
- Know the mechanism of nucleophilic acyl substitution reactions in both acidic and basic conditions, and how these reactions can be used to synthesize carboxylic acid derivatives
- Know the terms for specific examples: esterification, hydrolysis, saponification
- Know the relative reactivity of different carboxylic acid derivatives
- Know how long-chain carboxylic acids form micelles in aqueous solution
- Be able to recognize the principles of carbonyl chemistry in the context of the reactions of fatty acids and triacylglycerols
- Know the relative order of reactivity of different carboxylic acid derivatives
- Be aware of the acidity of alpha protons, and how abstraction of an alpha proton generates a carbonyl-containing nucleophile (leading to aldol condensation)
- Be aware of keto-enol tautomerism

10. Amines

- Know the rules for naming simple amines
- Be able to classify an amine as primary, secondary or tertiary
- Know the stereochemical and physical properties of amines
- Know how amines can form quaternary salts
- Know the factors affecting the basicity of amines, including aromatic amines
- Know the key ways to synthesize amines
- Know how amines act as nucleophiles in carbonyl reactions

cis-2-methylcyclohexanol:

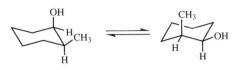

trans-2-methylcyclohexanol:

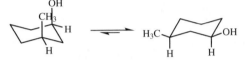

cis-3-methylcyclohexanol:

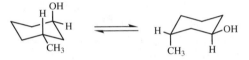

trans-3-methylcyclohexanol:

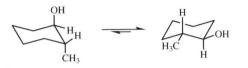

Choices **A** and **D** can only have one of its substituents occupy the equatorial position. Only choices **B** and **C** can adopt a conformation in which both substituents are equatorial, and this is the favored conformation for the compound. Choice **B** is therefore more stable than choice **A**, and choice **C** is more stable than choice **D**. We next need to decide which of the two diequatorial compounds is more stable: *trans*-2-methylcyclohexanol or *cis*-3-methylcyclohexanol. In *trans*-2-methylcyclohexanol, the substituents are on adjacent carbon atoms. When they both occupy the equatorial position, gauche interactions arise between the two. This is not as stable as in the case of *cis*-3-methylcyclohexanol, in which the two substituents are farther apart and hence no gauche interactions exist between them. Choice **C** is therefore the correct answer.

5. B

For the two compounds shown in the question stem, the antiperiplanar requirement for E2 to take place means that the chlorine (leaving group) needs to be in the axial position. We need to be careful in deducing the position of the alkyl substituents from the *cis/trans* relationship.

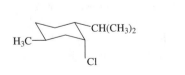

| Compound I | Compound II |

The conformation for each compound shown above is not necessarily the favored one. Rather, it is the conformation that the molecule must adopt if E2 were to occur, i.e., the one in which the chlorine is in the axial position. For example, in Compound I the isopropyl group is *cis* to the chlorine. When the chlorine is in the axial position, it *has* to occupy the equatorial position. Similarly, the methyl group two carbon atoms away from the chlorine has to be in the equatorial position based on its *cis/trans* relationship with chlorine.

The question stem asks us to determine two things: Which compound would undergo E2 more rapidly, and whether it leads to one or more products. As mentioned above, the conformation required for E2 is not necessarily the favored one. If, in order to undergo E2, the molecule must first adopt a conformation that is highly unfavorable, the reaction will be slow. This is the case for Compound II. With a "ring flip," the molecule can adopt another chair conformation in which the axial/equatorial positions of all substituents are reversed, leading to the following favored conformation in which all substituents are equatorial:

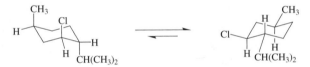

In other words, a molecule of Compound II must first adopt an unfavorable (strained) conformation before E2 can occur. This is expected to cause the reaction rate to decrease. In contrast, in its most stable conformation, Compound I is ready for E2 reaction: The chlorine is in the axial position and the two alkyl groups are equatorial. (It is not possible for all three substituents to occupy the equatorial position; a "ring flip" would result in two axial substituent groups and one equatorial substituent group.) The E2 reaction of Compound I is therefore expected to proceed more rapidly.

The remaining question we need to answer is: Does the E2 reaction of Compound I lead to one alkene product, or is there a possibility of multiple products? The base can abstract either one of the two protons antiperiplanar to the chlorine:

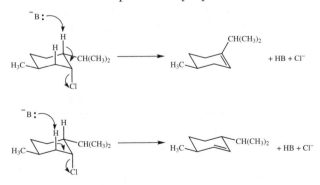

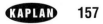

The reaction therefore leads to more than one product, and choice **B** is the correct answer.

6.   A

The chemistry of carbonyl compounds (ketones, aldehydes, carboxylic acids and their derivatives) is always an MCAT favorite. A thorough understanding of the principles behind the reactivity of these compounds and of the mechanisms of their common reactions is required. To answer this question, we need to have outside knowledge of the mechanism of ester hydrolysis, although the passage does describe the mechanism under both acidic and basic conditions for us. One of the key insights we need to gain is that every step of the acid-catalyzed hydrolysis of ester is a reversible equilibrium:

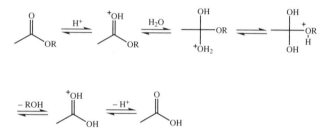

The reaction is completely reversible. Any individual ester molecule may go back and forth among the steps several times before forming the acid. Even then, if the product acid molecule encounters an R'OH molecule (an event of admittedly low probability since the solvent water molecules are much more plentiful), it may reform the ester.

In contrast, the base-promoted hydrolysis reaction does not yield the carboxylic acid, but the carboxylate anion, as described in the passage:

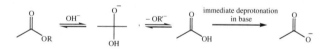

The reverse of the last deprotonation step is not expected to occur in basic conditions. In fact, when a base abstracts the proton from the carboxylic acid, it is irreversibly consumed and not recycled as a catalyst. (It is for this reason that purists refer to the reaction as "base-promoted" rather than "base-catalyzed.") Under basic conditions, then, the hydrolysis reaction is irreversible. Choice **A** is correct.

7.   B

Whenever an MCAT Organic Chemistry passage presents us with a complex, multistep reaction or synthesis scheme, we are likely to be asked to determine the outcome if one of the reagents used were isotopically labeled. This is one way the testmakers can see if we can follow what goes on in a reaction step by step and formulate a mechanism for that reaction (or particular steps in a reaction).

In this question, we are asked to determine where the O-18 isotope ends up if the compound shown in the question stem undergoes enzyme-catalyzed hydrolysis. The compound shown is an ester. Figure 1 illustrates the hydrolysis of an amide catalyzed by a serine protease, but the passage tells us that the enzyme also catalyzes the hydrolysis of esters. If we compare the structure given in the question to the amide in Figure 1, we see that the isotopically labeled oxygen plays the role of the nitrogen atom. The R and R' groups correspond as follows:

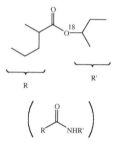

We are asked to determine where the isotopic label ends up. Again, by comparing the ester with the amide, we know that the answer can be found in Figure 1 by asking: What happens to the nitrogen atom of the amide? By examining the reaction, we know that the nitrogen atom is in the amine eliminated in Step 3. In other words, the C-N amide bond breaks, and the nitrogen-containing portion grabs a proton and leaves. If we apply this to the ester, we expect the C-O ester linkage to break, and the oxygen-containing portion to grab a proton and leave. What is the resulting molecule? An alcohol. More specifically, the oxygen will be incorporated into the following alcohol molecule:

$$HO-\overset{18}{}$$

Choice **B** is therefore correct.

Choice **A** is incorrect. In order for the carboxylic acid molecule in the product to bear the isotopically labeled oxygen atom, the label should come from either the carbonyl oxygen of the ester, or the water molecule in Step 3. Choice **C** is incorrect because no water molecule is generated during the reaction. Choice **D** is incorrect because we can see that the serine residue keeps its oxygen atom throughout the reaction.

8.   C

This question demonstrates the importance of knowing the rules of nomenclature of organic compounds for the MCAT. We cannot answer the question correctly without knowing the structure of N-propylbutanamide, as shown in the following diagram:

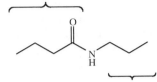

four-carbon carboxylic acid derivative

propyl group attached to N

If we compare this structure to the generic one shown in Figure 1, R and R' are both propyl groups. (R + carbonyl carbon = 4 carbons, hence <u>butan</u>amide.) In step 3, then, the amine that is formed and eliminated from the enzyme-substrate complex must have the formula $NH_2CH_2CH_2CH_3$. This is 1-propanamine. The R group ends up as part of a carboxylic acid molecule at the end of step 5. If R is a propyl group, the acid must therefore be butanoic acid. Hence, choice **C** is correct.

9.   C
This is a very challenging question because it calls for both sophisticated reasoning as well as an intimate knowledge of the principles of reactivity. In an earlier question, we concluded that ester hydrolysis is reversible in acidic but irreversible in basic conditions. One might expect the same to be true of amide hydrolysis. But according to the question stem here, this is not true: In fact, we are told, amide hydrolysis is irreversible in both acidic and basic conditions. The choices present us with some factors that may contribute to the explanation and we are asked to identify the one that is NOT expected to play a role. In this case it is best to evaluate each choice in turn.

Choice **A** states that the amine product becomes protonated at low pH. This statement is true because amines are weakly basic. In acidic (low pH) conditions, we expect the nitrogen to be protonated, forming a quaternary ammonium salt. Does this fact provide an explanation? Yes: In order for the hydrolysis reaction to be reversed (for the amide to reform), at some point an amine must act as a nucleophile and attack the carbonyl carbon of the acid, and subsequently displace a water molecule. This cannot happen if the nitrogen atom has no nucleophilic electron pair, which is the case at low pH. Choice **A** therefore DOES play a role in the irreversibility of the reaction and cannot be the correct answer.

Choice **B** states that at low pH, the nitrogen atom in the tetrahedral intermediate favors being protonated. This is also a true statement, as we know that the nitrogen atom is basic. Indeed, the protonation of the nitrogen is a crucial step in the hydrolysis of an amide, as it creates a good leaving group:

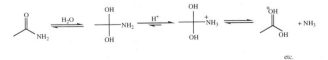

etc.

Protonation is more likely to occur at the nitrogen than it is at either oxygen atom, so the hydrolysis product forms more easily. Protonation of an oxygen would create a good water leaving group, whose departure would lead to the original amide. However, this is precisely what needs to occur if the hydrolysis is to be reversible. This is not expected to happen easily.

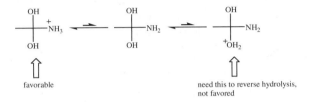

Choice **B**, then, also helps explain why amide hydrolysis is not reversible in acidic conditions, and therefore cannot be the right choice.

Choice **C** states that at high pH, amide hydrolysis involves the elimination of the strongly basic NH_2^- as leaving group. This is again a correct statement, as indicated in the passage, and as can be verified by envisioning the mechanism for amide hydrolysis in basic conditions. After the nucleophilic attack by hydroxide, the tetrahedral intermediate has the following structure:

Since the solution is basic, there is no proton source to protonate the nitrogen. In order for hydrolysis to proceed, the C-N bond must break, and this can only occur with NH_2^- as the leaving group. Since it is strongly basic, it is not a good leaving group. (In fact, NH_2^- abstracts a proton from a nearby molecule to form ammonia either concurrently with or immediately after elimination.) It is for this reason that harsh conditions are needed to carry out amide hydrolysis in base. Amides are considered "kinetically stable" in base.

This observation, however, does not help to explain why amide hydrolysis is irreversible. It simply tells us that it may be difficult to get the reaction going in the forward (hydrolysis) direction. Choice **C** is therefore the correct answer.

We can consider choice **D** for completeness. Choice **D** states that at high pH, the carboxylate ion does not possess a good leaving group. This is accurate. In base, the hydrolysis product is the carboxylate anion, just as in ester hydrolysis. For the same reason that ester hydrolysis is irreversible in base, this statement provides an explanation to the irreversibility of amide hydrolysis in base.

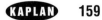

10. B

An acyl group has the following structure:

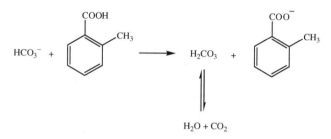

An acyl-enzyme intermediate is therefore one in which the carbonyl carbon is bonded to the enzyme on the other end. Such a structure is formed in Step 2 where the –COR group is bonded to the enzyme at the serine 195 residue.

Step 1 leads to the formation of a tetrahedral intermediate. Step 3 involves the elimination of the amine. Step 4 actually breaks the acyl-enzyme complex to form another tetrahedral intermediate.

11. D

An MCAT passage that presents an extraction sequence is usually accompanied by questions testing our understanding of the rationale behind specific steps. Often, how the acid-base properties of a compound affect its solubility is the key to the question. In step 1, a weak base (bicarbonate ion, HCO_3^-) was added to the mixture. It will cause a relatively strong acid to deprotonate, converting it into its conjugate base. If the conjugate base is charged it will migrate into the aqueous layer where it preferentially dissolves, leaving the other nonacidic (or less acidic) organic compounds behind in the organic layer. This is the principle behind the separation. Among the four compounds shown, 2-methylbenzoic acid is the strongest acid and is expected to be the one extracted in step 1. The bicarbonate ion causes it to deprotonate, and the carboxylate conjugate base dissolves in the aqueous layer. The HCl that was subsequently added reformed the acid. Before the addition of HCl, therefore, the predominant form of Compound A (which again we can conclude is 2-methylbenzoic acid) is the carboxylate ion, answer choice **A**.

The other choices either are not the conjugate base of a strong acid, or will not be extracted into the aqueous layer. Choice **A**, an amine salt, is the conjugate *acid* of an amine, not the conjugate base of something. Choice **B**, an amine, IS the conjugate base of a relatively strong acid, R_3NH^+. However, R_3NH^+, as a charged species, is already water-soluble. Addition of the bicarbonate would cause the formation of the *neutral* amine conjugate base. The neutral amine is expected to be less soluble in water than the conjugate acid, so it is not a likely method of extracting an amine. Choice **C** is the conjugate base of phenol, which is not as strong an acid as carboxylic acid. It will take the much more basic hydroxide ion in step 2 to deprotonate phenol.

12. A

Pressure buildup within the funnel needs to be avoided since it may cause the funnel to explode. This is something we need to watch out for whenever gas may be generated. This question is therefore essentially asking us to identify the step in the procedure that leads to the generation of gas. The only step in which a gas is created is step 1, in which bicarbonate abstracts a proton from an acid:

The carbonic acid (H_2CO_3) formed establishes an equilibrium with carbon dioxide, which may escape from solution. (This results in the fizzing usually observed.) The generation of gas is the reason why we are usually instructed to shake the separatory funnel gently and vent often after each agitation.

13. C

The MCAT expects students to be familiar with different techniques used to characterize compounds, and be able to identify the technique that is most appropriate in a given situation. In this question we are asked how we could tell if the solution containing Compound C (the solution obtained after step 4) also contains a fifth, unknown compound. In other words, we are looking for a technique that will tell us how many distinct components there are in the mixture. Thin-layer chromatography (TLC), choice **C**, is the appropriate technique: The number of components in the mixture will be revealed as the number of spots in the final chromatogram. (Different compounds will migrate up the plate at different rates based on their polarity and be assigned different R_f values.)

Choice **A**, nuclear magnetic resonance, is a very useful technique in deducing the structure of a compound because it reveals the types of protons present in the molecule and how many of each proton type there are. However, if we supply a sample that actually contains two compounds, the spectrum will not inform us of this fact. This is also true of choices **B** and **D**, IR spectroscopy and mass spectrometry. In particular, mass spectrometry causes the sample to break up into charged fragments, a step that essentially eliminates all information as to where the fragments may have come from.

14. C

Benzylamine has the formula $C_6H_5CH_2NH_2$. Even if we could not identify the structure, we should at least be able to infer from its name the presence of an amine group, which is weakly basic. Its extraction can be accomplished by first adding an acid, then isolating the aqueous portion.

The addition of acid protonates the base, causing it to form the cationic conjugate acid $C_6H_5CH_2NH_3^+$. The cation dissolves in the aqueous layer because of the favorable solvation interactions by water molecules. The original neutral compound can be obtained by the introduction of another base which abstracts a proton from the conjugate acid. This is precisely what occurs in step 3. HCl protonates 4-methylaniline, which in its conjugate acid form will dissolve in the aqueous layer. Addition of NaOH causes the conjugate acid to deprotonate and yield the neutral aniline back. (Compound B is therefore 4-methylaniline.) Since benzylamine contains the same amine functional group, if it were present in the mixture it would also be extracted in the same step.

15. D

To answer this question correctly we need to be able to do two things: Identify which proton type the compounds have in common, and then determine the chemical shift of this proton type. On the MCAT, students are expected to know the characteristic shifts of different proton types.

The only protons that all four compounds have in common are aryl protons: protons directly attached to an aromatic ring (this is the only type of proton that naphthalene possesses). Aromatic protons give proton-NMR signals with a chemical shift closest to that listed in choice **D**.

The chemical shift given in choice **A** is characteristic of methyl protons in saturated hydrocarbons. The chemical shift of choice **B** is characteristic of acetylenic protons ($-C\equiv C\text{-}\mathbf{H}$), alpha protons in ketones ($-\mathbf{CH}COR$), and benzylic protons ($Ar\text{-}\mathbf{CH}\text{-}$, e.g., the methyl protons on 2-methylbenzoic acid, 4-methylaniline, and *p*-cresol). The chemical shift of choice **C** is characteristic of vinylic protons ($=\mathbf{CH}R$).

16. D

One of the skills tested on the MCAT is our ability to interpret the results of an experiment. This question asks us to determine what conclusions can be drawn about the structure of (+)-glucose given the fact that when oxidized by nitric acid, the resulting dicarboxylic acid is optically active. To arrive at the correct answer, we have to be able to visualize very concretely what happens to an aldohexose in the oxidation reaction.

First, we notice that all the compounds shown in Figure 1 are optically active. No plane of symmetry is possible since at one end of each molecule is an aldehyde group while at the other end is a primary alcohol group. However, we are told in the passage that nitric acid oxidation converts both these groups into the carboxyl group. Now that the two ends of the molecule are the same, there is a possibility of symmetry, and hence of optical inactivity. Those

aldohexoses in which the arrangement of –OH vs. –H groups in the stereocenters is symmetric will be optically inactive after nitric acid oxidation.

We are told that after (+)-glucose has been oxidized by nitric acid oxidation, the resulting dicarboxylic acid is still optically active. That means that even with the two ends of the molecule now identical, there is still no plane of symmetry in the molecule. Hence, we can conclude that the arrangement of –OH versus –H groups in the stereocenters is not symmetric in (+)-glucose to begin with. We can eliminate from the eight structures any compound with such a symmetric arrangement from consideration. This is compound VII:

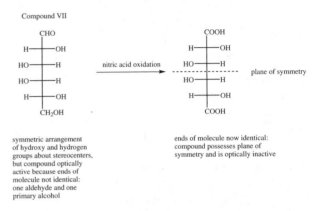

Compound VII

symmetric arrangement of hydroxy and hydrogen groups about stereocenters, but compound optically active because ends of molecule not identical: one aldehyde and one primary alcohol

ends of molecule now identical: compound possesses plane of symmetry and is optically inactive

(Incidentally, we can also eliminate Compound I as a possible candidate for the structure of (+)-glucose from the same reasoning. The aldaric acid formed from either Compound I or Compound VII is a meso compound: It possesses stereocenters, but because a plane of symmetry exists for the molecule, it is optically inactive.)

The other compounds listed in the answer choices (Compounds IV, V, and VI), as well as Compounds II, III, and VIII, still remain as possibilities for glucose because they would all generate optically active aldaric acids upon nitric acid oxidation. For example, compound IV generates the following aldaric acid:

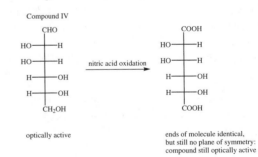

Compound IV

optically active

ends of molecule identical, but still no plane of symmetry: compound still optically active

17. C

This question tests us on our ability to apply our knowledge of stereochemistry to monosaccharides. D- and L-sugars of the same name are enantiomers, i.e.,

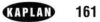

nonsuperimposable mirror images. Enantiomers differ in the configuration of every stereocenter. We can construct the enantiomer of L-gulose and match it with the compounds shown in Figure 1:

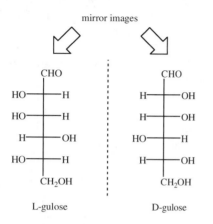

L-gulose   D-gulose

We can see that the structure of D-gulose is identical to that of Compound V.

Among the wrong answer choices, notice that Compound IV differs from L-gulose in the configuration of the highest-numbered stereocenter only. This does not make it the enantiomer of L-gulose because the configuration about every stereocenter has to be different in order for two compounds to be enantiomers. Instead, Compound IV and L-gulose are diastereomers. Indeed, Compounds III and VI (the other incorrect choices) are both diastereomers of L-gulose, of D-gulose, of Compound IV, and of each other.

18. D
Some fundamental knowledge of carbohydrate terminology is needed for the MCAT. A ketohexose is a six-carbon (hence *hex*) monosaccharide with a ketone (RCOR') rather than an aldehyde (RCHO) functionality (hence *keto*). In other words, the carbonyl carbon should be bonded to (non-hydrogen) alkyl groups on both sides. Only choice **D** satisfies both criteria.

Choice **A** is an aldohexose (six carbon atoms, but aldehyde functionality). Indeed, it is identical to Compound V in Figure 1, with the aldehyde group drawn explicitly. Choice **B** is a ketose, but only has five carbons. It is therefore a ketopentose. Choice **C** is also a ketose, but has seven carbons.

19. B
The passage indicates that the Kiliani-Fischer synthesis lengthens the carbon chain by one carbon at the aldehyde group, creating a new stereogenic center. In other words, the products are as follows:

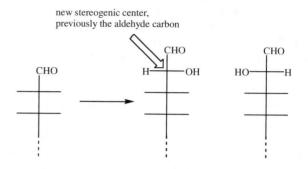

new stereogenic center, previously the aldehyde carbon

Notice that the rest of the molecule remains the same, so the two products are NOT enantiomers, but diastereomers that differ in the configuration of only one of the stereocenters (the newly created one).

We are told in the passage that when Fischer carried out the synthesis on an aldopentose, he obtained a mixture (+)-glucose and (+)-mannose. The two compounds must therefore differ only in the configuration about the first stereocenter (C2, the carbon atom immediately after the aldehyde group). This is true only of Compounds III and IV among the pairs given in the choices. In fact, we can conclude that (−)-arabinose must have the following structure:

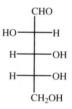

Choice **A**, Compounds II and III, differ in the configuration of C2 and C3. Choice **C**, Compounds V and VII, differ in the configuration of C3 only, not C2. Choice **D**, Compounds VI and VII, differ in the configuration of C2 and C3.

20. A
One of the properties of carbohydrates that we need to be aware of is the possibility of cyclization of some monosaccharides. In solution, aldohexoses tend to undergo cyclization to form a compound with a stable six-membered ring. This is accomplished by having the hydroxy group on the C5 atom attack the aldehyde carbon:

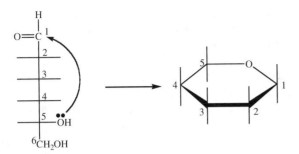

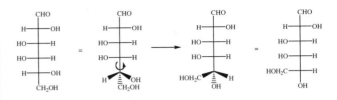

In this question, we are asked to identify the cyclic form of a compound whose linear structure is shown. To accomplish this task, it is of crucial importance to keep track of which carbon atom ends up where. One of the groups attached to C5 will be the –CH$_2$OH group. In other words, C6 is not part of the ring. In this question, we need to determine the orientation of the various –OH and –H groups, which is quite challenging. However, we can compare the relative configurations of the stereocenters in the linear versus the cyclic form. If we study Compound VII, we can see that C3 and C4 have their hydroxy groups pointing in the same direction, which is opposite to that of C2. In the cyclic structure, then, we look for the compound in which the hydroxy group on C2 points one way, while the hydroxy groups on C3 and C4 point the other way. This is choice **A.**

The "squiggly line" depicting the bond between C1 and its hydroxy group indicates that we are not interested in its orientation. We will get a mixture of both configurations at that stereocenter from the cyclization reaction. The two products are the α- and β-anomers.

Notice that this reasoning is adequate only because the answer choices do not ask us to choose between the following two compounds:

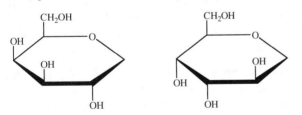

The structure on the left is choice **A.** The structure on the right (fortunately) does not appear among the answer choices. If it had, then we would have to determine how the orientation of the –CH$_2$OH group is related to the orientation of the hydroxy groups. This can be done by mentally rotating the C4-C5 bond in the linear molecule:

The –CH$_2$OH group therefore should point in the same direction as the hydroxy groups on C3 and C4, thus confirming that choice **A** is correct.

Choice **B** corresponds to the cyclic structure of Compound IV. Choice **C** corresponds to the cyclic form of Compound VI. Choice **D** is the cyclic form of Compound VIII.

21. B

This question tests whether we can apply the definition of a conjugate acid-base pair, but more importantly, it tests our knowledge of nomenclature of some nitrogen-containing compounds. If the product of Step 3 is the conjugate acid of something (whose identity we are trying to determine), then that "something" must be the conjugate base of the product of Step 3. The most acidic proton in the product of Step 3 is the one on the nitrogen atom. The question, then, is asking us to identify the name of the following functional group:

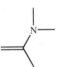

The compound contains an alkene functional group. One of the sp^2-hybridized carbon atoms is bonded to a nitrogen atom. This species is an enamine, so choice **B** is correct.

The structures of the incorrect answer choices are as follows:

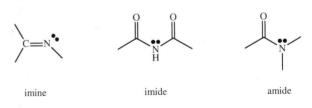

imine   imide   amide

22. D

This question takes us a little beyond the scope of the passage itself and asks us to determine what happens when the product of the reaction is subjected to certain reaction conditions (heat). MCAT questions do sometimes use a compound mentioned in the passage as a springboard for questions on aspects of organic chemistry not directly relevant to the passage itself. The final product of the reaction is a β-hydroxyketone: There is a hydroxy group bonded to the carbon atom that is beta to the carbonyl

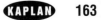

carbon. In other words, in addition to the carbonyl functionality, it also acts as an alcohol. When heated, therefore, the compound, like many other alcohols, will undergo dehydration, a reaction in which a water molecule is eliminated. The generic alcohol dehydration is an acid-catalyzed reaction:

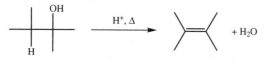

In this particular case, the driving force is the formation of a carbon-carbon pi bond that can be conjugated with the carbonyl pi bond. The double bond, therefore, has to be between the alpha and beta carbons.

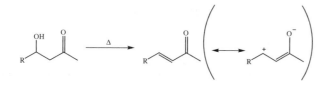

Choices **A** and **B** are incorrect because heating alone is not sufficient to cause the compound to decompose into two carbonyl compounds. The products resemble those we might obtain from oxidative cleavage of alkenes, but the starting compound is not an alkene and the conditions for oxidative cleavage are not present. Choice **C** is incorrect because the hydroxy group should no longer be a part of the molecule after dehydration.

23. D

This question asks us to deduce the conditions needed for Step 1 to proceed as indicated in the passage. It is a challenging question asking us to engage in relatively sophisticated reasoning based on the acid-base properties of the compounds involved. Step 1 involves the nucleophilic attack of the nitrogen in proline on the carbonyl carbon of acetone. The conditions must NOT be acidic. If they were, the nitrogen atom would be protonated and there would not be a lone pair of electrons available for nucleophilic attack. The medium must therefore be neutral or slightly basic to ensure that the nitrogen does not form a quaternary salt. However, immediately after the addition has taken place, we would obtain an alkoxide ion. The product of Step 1 as shown can only be accomplished by protonating the alkoxide in acidic conditions. This protonation step is necessary in order to get the dehydration in the next step to occur. In fact, further protonation (converting the hydroxy group into a water molecule) is necessary to create the leaving group. Choice **D** is therefore correct.

24. B

The MCAT may ask us to evaluate proposed hypotheses in light of information presented in the passage to test our

critical thinking skills. This question is essentially asking us to account for the enantioselectivity of the illustrated reaction. The stereogenic center in the β-hydroxyketone is created in Step 4 when the aldehyde adds to the proline-acetone complex. The transition state of Step 4 is shown in the passage. As mentioned in the passage, the transition state is a tricyclic complex, and one of the three rings is a six-membered ring involving the aldehyde. Notice that the R group is in the favored, equatorial position. In other words, the aldehyde adopts the more stable orientation relative to the complex, and it is this orientation preference that leads to the predominant creation of one enantiomer. In order to create the other enantiomer, the R and H will have to be swapped in the aldehyde. (i.e., the aldehyde will have to be rotated 180° about an axis going through the carbonyl bond.) That, however, will lead to higher strain in the transition state, as the R group will be in the axial position.

Choice **A** is incorrect because we are not adding different halves of a molecule across the double bond, so the Markovnikov versus anti-Markovnikov designation is irrelevant. Choice **C** is incorrect. A general principle in organic synthesis is that we will never be able to create net optical activity using only optically inactive reagents. In other words, in order to create an enantiomer without its mirror image, there must be some chiral environment or reagents introduced at some point. If we started with a racemic mixture of proline, the final product would be a racemic mixture of the R and S isomers of the β-hydroxyketone. Choice **D** is incorrect because the aldehyde is achiral. It does not have an enantiomer.

25. A

The MCAT expects students to identify the names of processes and transformations that occur in the course of a reaction. For this question, we are asked to determine which of the four processes does NOT occur. In other words, to eliminate an answer choice as incorrect, we should be able to see an example of it in the reaction.

The two carbonyl compounds involved in the reaction are a ketone and an aldehyde. Neither possesses a good leaving group. So no nucleophilic acyl substitution reaction is possible. The general scheme for a nucleophilic acyl substitution reaction is shown below:

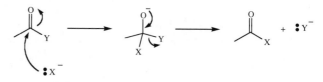

(The last step of the reaction is similar to the second step of a nucleophilic acyl substitution reaction under acidic conditions. The carbon-oxygen pi bond is formed as the proline acts as a leaving group and departs. However, the new carbonyl oxygen has never been part of a carbonyl compound. Instead, it comes from the water molecule that adds to the compound in Step 5, so the reaction is not a nucleophilic acyl substitution reaction.)

Choice **B** is incorrect because it does occur in Step 1: The nitrogen acts as a nucleophile and attacks the carbonyl carbon. Choice **C** is incorrect because addition to an alkene does occur in Step 4. The pi electrons of the C=C bond in the enamine are used to form the sigma bond to the aldehyde. Choice **D** is incorrect because Steps 5 and 6 together constitute a hydrolysis reaction: A molecule is broken apart via the addition of a water molecule.

26. A

If we have very strong outside knowledge (possibly beyond the scope of what the MCAT requires), we can answer the question without any help from the passage. But the question can be answered with an understanding and synthesis of different components of the passage.

Hydrogenation is mentioned in the first two tests described in the passage. It is imperative to pay close attention to the different results in the two cases. In the first test, we are told that hydrogenation of the unknown over Pd/C yielded stearic acid. From the condensed structural formula given for stearic acid, we should be able to tell that the alkyl portion of the acid is completely saturated; i.e., there are no carbon-carbon double or triple bonds. In Test 2, with the use of Lindlar's catalyst, only two molar equivalents of hydrogen were absorbed. In other words, only two pi bonds were saturated. The results of these two tests by themselves do not suggest any immediately obvious difference, and in fact they may have led to the exact same compound. The question to ask, then, is do the two tests actually yield the same compound? Is stearic acid obtained by saturating two pi bonds? To answer this we need to turn to the possible structures of the compounds given at the end of the passage. Both structures contain two carbon-carbon triple bonds and one carbon-carbon double bond. To convert the unknown into stearic acid requires the saturation of every carbon-carbon pi bond in the compound and would therefore require the absorption of five molar equivalents of hydrogen. (Recall that a triple bond contains two pi bonds and a double bond contains one pi bond.) Absorption of two molar equivalents of hydrogen (using Lindlar's catalyst) would still leave some pi bonds intact. What functionality do we have two of in the unknown? Triple bonds. It is therefore reasonable to assume that each triple bond is converted into a double bond, leaving a product containing three C=C bonds. Choice **A** is therefore correct. The situation is summarized for each of the two proposed structures in the diagram that follows:

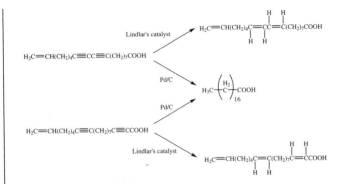

Choice **B** is not supported by evidence in the passage and can also be rejected because of its implausibility: Saturating a carbon-oxygen double bond (i.e., converting a carbonyl functionality into a hydroxy group) requires only one molar equivalent of hydrogen. Choice **C** is also unsupported and implausible: If we could determine the identity of the end product and if we knew the degree of unsaturation of the unknown, then there is no reason why quantitative measurement of hydrogen absorbed is not possible. Choice **D** is incorrect because hydrogenation reactions are by definition reduction reactions.

27. A

In Test 3, the unknown is oxidized in $KMnO_4$. We are told that three of the products are dicarboxylic acids, and we are asked to determine the identity of the remaining product. We can examine the possible structures of the unknown (given at the end of the passage) and try to determine the effect of oxidation by $KMnO_4$. In general, $KMnO_4$ will cleave a carbon-carbon double and triple bond and convert each carbon on the end into a carboxylic acid functionality (after acid work-up). (Under mild conditions use of $KMnO_4$ on an alkene may lead instead to the formation of diols; i.e., only the pi bond in the double bond will be broken. But the passage already indicates that carboxylic acids are formed.) If the unknown had the first of the two possible structures, the three dicarboxylic acids would have been obtained in the following manner:

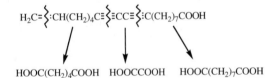

At this point we realize that the question can be rephrased as: What happens to the terminal methylene group upon oxidation? That product is the one species that is not a dicarboxylic acid. If our outside knowledge is strong, we can arrive at carbon dioxide as the correct answer immediately. But even if we are not aware of this, we may still have been able to eliminate the other choices. Our first intuition may be to treat the methylene group no differently: The carbon atom would become a carboxylic acid functional group:

$$H_2C = \bigg\{ = \quad \xrightarrow{[O]} \quad \overset{\overset{\textstyle O}{\textstyle \|}}{\text{HCOH}}$$

or maybe even

$$\overset{\overset{\textstyle O}{\textstyle \|}}{\text{HOCOH}}$$

However, neither structure is among the answer choices.

We therefore have to resort to elimination. Choice **B** can be rejected because potassium permanganate cannot generate an extra carbon. The number of carbon atoms in each species is determined by the structure of the original compound (where the double and triple bonds occur). Choice **C** may be harder to reject, but we may surmise that if the reagent is capable of oxidizing all the other functionalities "all the way" to a carboxylic acid (with three C-O) bonds, it is strange to halt the oxidation of the terminal methylene group at the alcohol stage. In other words, we would expect the species to be more oxidized. Choice **D** can be rejected because it is not an oxidation product but a reduction product. After we have tentatively rejected the other answer choices, we may be able to justify to ourselves why carbon dioxide is a reasonable choice. It is as oxidized as one can get (consistent with the production of dicarboxylic acids), and stoichiometrically it works:

$$H_2C = \bigg\{ = \quad \xrightarrow{[O]} \quad CO_2 + H_2O$$

28. D

The question asks us to identify the one piece of information that can be deduced based on Test 1, but cannot be deduced based on Test 5. The results of Test 5 need not contradict the information, and indeed, it should not, since the tests are conducted on the same compound. So, the results of Test 5 should be unrelated to the property established by Test 1.

Test 1 indicates that upon hydrogenation, the unknown was converted into stearic acid, whose condensed structural formula is then given. Test 5 indicates that the unknown only has one –COOH group. The results of the two tests certainly do not contradict each other (and as mentioned above, they had better not!). In other words, the fact that the unknown yields stearic acid upon hydrogenation implies whatever is stated in the correct choice. However, the fact that it has one –COOH group does not in and of itself enable us to say that whatever is stated in the correct choice is true. What remains to be done now is to evaluate each answer choice in turn.

Choice **A** states that the unknown contains unsaturated carbon atoms. This is an incorrect choice because it is necessarily true given the result of Test 5: The carbonyl carbon of a carboxylic acid functional group is unsaturated. Choice **B** states that the unknown is not capable of *cis/trans* isomerism. *Cis/trans* isomerism can occur if the unknown contains a C=C bond, *and* if each carbon of the double bond is attached two different groups. Test 1 tells us that the compound is unsaturated, but by itself it doesn't tell us if the compound contains C=C bonds (as opposed to the unsaturation arising solely from triple bonds), nor does it tell us what groups are attached to the double-bonded carbon atoms if they exist. Choice **B** is therefore not inferable from Test 1. Choice **C** states that the unknown contains an acidic hydrogen. This is inferable from *both* tests, so cannot be the correct choice. Choice **D**, by the process of elimination, must be correct. From the condensed structural formula of stearic acid, we can tell that the alkyl portion is straight-chained (seventeen carbons in a row followed by a –COOH group). The unknown must therefore also not be branched, since hydrogenation by itself does not rearrange the carbon skeleton. The fact that the unknown is unbranched is therefore inferable from Test 1. However, it is not inferable from Test 5, which has nothing to do with the alkyl portion. Just because it contains one –COOH group reveals nothing about what the alkyl portion might be like.

29. C

The question asks us to determine the one property that will set stearic acid and the unknown apart. From the answer choices, we can tell that the property can be based on either IR spectrum, NMR spectrum, or boiling point. The correct answer must therefore apply to one of the two compounds. Incorrect answer choices will be true of both compounds or of neither compound.

What is needed from the passage is an awareness of the structural differences between stearic acid and the unknown. The unknown, unlike stearic acid, has carbon-carbon double and triple bonds. The distinguishing feature is therefore expected to hinge on the presence (or absence) of these unsaturated bonds. With this in mind, we can evaluate the answer choices. Choice **A** refers to a singlet in the proton NMR spectrum between 10 and 12 ppm. This chemical shift corresponds to the proton of a carboxylic acid group, which is present in both compounds. This feature therefore cannot be used to distinguish between the two. Choice **B** refers to a strong and broad IR absorption from 2500 to 3400 cm^{-1}. This band is characteristic of an O-H bond, which again is present on both compounds. So this too cannot be used to distinguish between them. Choice **C** refers to the absence of any IR stretches around 2200 cm^{-1}. This is where a C≡C bond is expected to absorb, so its absence would signify that the compound is stearic acid and not the unknown, which we know contains triple bonds. Choice **C** is therefore the correct answer. Finally, choice **D** can be rejected because both compounds, being carboxylic acids, will have higher boiling points than the corresponding alcohol. In fact, the alcohol listed in the answer choice has one fewer carbon atom, making its boiling point even lower.

30. C
Determining the isomeric relationship between two compounds is an MCAT favorite. Geometric isomers are isomers arising from the arrangement of groups around a double bond. While the structures do both contain a C=C bond, the fact that one carbon is attached to two hydrogen atoms (two identical groups) precludes the possibility of geometric isomers. So choice **A** is incorrect. Choice **B** is also incorrect because diastereomers are either geometric isomers (rejected as a possibility) or stereoisomers with multiple chiral centers that are not enantiomers of each other. The structures proposed do not contain any chiral center, so they cannot be diastereomers. Choice **C** is correct: They differ in the connectivity of the atoms. In one case, the carboxyl group is attached to a chain of seven saturated carbon atoms; in the other case, the carboxyl group is directly bonded to an *sp*-hybridized carbon. Choice **D** is incorrect because the two structures have the same molecular formula and are therefore isomers of each other.

31. C
Questions asking for the number of stereogenic centers in a compound are a perennial MCAT favorite. A stereogenic center, also referred to on the MCAT as a stereocenter or a chiral center, is (usually) a carbon atom bonded to four different groups. (Nitrogen and some other heteroatoms can also act as stereocenters if the arrangement of groups about the atom leads to distinct, nonsuperimposable mirror images.) The stereocenters of lovastatin, whose structure is shown in Equation 2, are labeled with an asterisk in the diagram below.

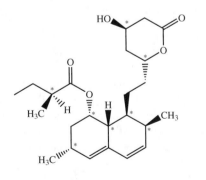

There are a total of eight stereocenters. Notice that we always need to keep in mind that hydrogen atoms needed to saturate the carbon atoms are not always indicated explicitly in chemical structures. However, if there are two such "implied hydrogens" attached to a carbon atom, that carbon atom cannot possibly be a stereocenter because it will not be bonded to four different groups. For this reason, the two carbon atoms labeled below are not stereocenters:

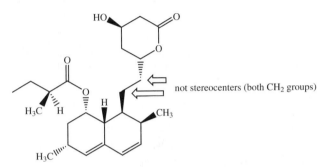

not stereocenters (both CH₂ groups)

Besides this issue of "implied hydrogen atoms," the other pitfall for questions like this arises in the case of a multicyclic compound. In the diagram below, the structure on the left has no stereocenters, but the structure on the right has two stereocenters. Each of the atoms labeled with an asterisk is bonded to four distinct groups: The "bridge," a hydrogen atom, one half of the six-membered ring with the carbonyl group, and the other half of the six-membered ring without the carbonyl group. (In the structure on the left, the two halves of the six-membered ring are identical, so the four groups are not distinct.)

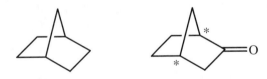

32. A
An MCAT Organic Chemistry passage that presents a new reaction may often be accompanied by questions in which we need to apply the reaction to a new set of reactants and determine the product(s). To answer this question, we need to first of all determine the structure of cyclopentadiene and then apply Equation 1 to the situation in which one molecule of cyclopentadiene acts as the diene while another molecule acts as the dienophile.

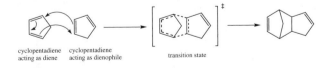

cyclopentadiene acting as diene   cyclopentadiene acting as dienophile   transition state

This is the structure shown in choice **A**. Even if we had not been able to visualize how the spatial relationships between the bonds evolve over the course of the reaction, we could have eliminated the other answer choices by some reasoning and by close examination of Equation 1. In Equation 1, we see that the diene and the dienophile join to form a six-membered ring, with a double bond in the position between the two double bonds in the original diene. Furthermore, we go from three double bonds (one from the dienophile and two from the diene) to one double bond in the product. In the case with two molecules of cyclopentadiene, however, we start off with an extra double bond: The dienophile itself contains two double bonds, one of which does not participate in the reaction. The number of double bonds in the product, then, is expected to be two. This enables us to eliminate choice **D**. Furthermore, we know that the second double bond in the product should not be part of the six-membered ring; i.e., the six-membered ring should only contain the one double bond that forms as a result of the reaction. Choice **B** can therefore be eliminated. Finally, choice **C** can be eliminated because the six-membered ring does not contain any double bond. The structure shown has both double bonds as part of a five-membered ring, which contradicts the reaction as illustrated in Equation 1.

33. C

In this question, we are asked to determine where an isotopic label ends up after the reaction. This can be a very challenging question as the reaction, as illustrated in Equation 3, contains very little that can help us orient ourselves spatially to see how the two compounds join to form the bicyclic compound. However, we can keep track of certain functional groups. By examining where the $-OCH_3$, $-COCH_3$ and $-CH_3$ groups end up in the bicyclic compound, we can deduce how the molecule is "put together":

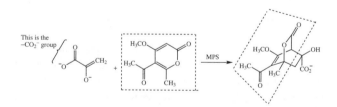

With the spatial relationships established, we can see that the radiolabeled oxygen in the question stem becomes the oxygen in the hydroxy group of the bicyclic compound. Choice **C** is therefore correct. The following diagram illustrates how the electrons are actually shifted around in the reaction.

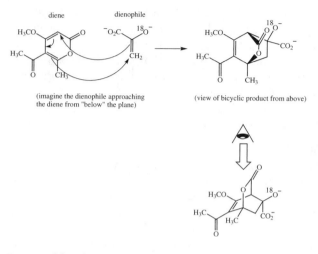

(imagine the dienophile approaching the diene from "below" the plane)

(view of bicyclic product from above)

Presumably the oxygen is protonated during an acid "work-up" step to create the hydroxy group.

34. B

The question is essentially asking us to identify the one compound that will not participate in a Diels-Alder reaction. The choices are meant to act as analogs of the 2-pyrone shown in Equation 3. As the passage states, the Diels-Alder reaction involves the addition of an alkene (acting as a dienophile) to a conjugated diene. In addition, as can be deduced from examining the reaction shown in Equation 3, the 2-pyrone acts as the diene. In other words, the analogs must be conjugated dienes. A diene is conjugated if the pi electrons can be delocalized across the double bonds. In other words, we should be able to draw resonance structures for the compound in which the pi electrons are shifted around:

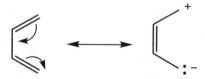

The compound shown in choice **B** is not a conjugated diene: The two carbon-carbon double bonds are separated by sp^3-hybridized atoms and the pi electrons are therefore not delocalized. It therefore cannot react with a dienophile to yield a Diels-Alder adduct.

35. D

The question is asking us to identify the process that will convert lovastatin as it appears in Equation 2 to the structure shown in the question stem. Focusing on the portion of the molecule that has undergone change, we are essentially asked to determine the name for the following transformation:

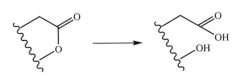

The original functionality is a (cyclic) ester, with the formula –COOR. The functionalities after the transformation are a carboxylic acid and an alcohol. The process is therefore one of ester hydrolysis.

Choices **A** and **B**, oxidation and reduction, are incorrect because the number of carbon-oxygen bonds has not changed. Recall that oxidation of an organic compound implies forming more bonds between carbon and oxygen atoms (or between carbon and some other electronegative heteroatoms like nitrogen and chlorine), while the reduction of an organic compound implies forming more C-H bonds. The carbonyl carbon in the ester has three C-O bonds (one double and one single); the same is true in the carboxylic acid product. Choice **C**, ozonolysis, refers to the formation of carbonyl compounds by breaking a carbon-carbon double bond. The general ozonolysis scheme is as follows:

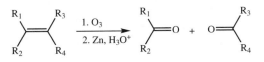

Discrete Questions

36. B
The molecular formula of a compound indicates the number of atoms of each element in one molecule of the substance. The molecular formula for glucose, for example, is $C_6H_{12}O_6$. However, the molecular formula does not provide full information on the structure of the molecule or on what functional groups it contains. Drawing the structure out is not always feasible. Hence, organic chemists sometimes make use of condensed structural formulas to convey information on the structure. The MCAT expects test takers to be able to interpret condensed structural formulas.

The condensed structural formula given in the question corresponds to the following compound:

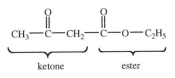

The compound therefore has both a ketone and an ester functionality. Since only ester appears as a choice, choice **B** is the correct answer.

Ethers, choice **A**, have the general formula ROR'. A condensed structural formula, for example, may look like $CH_3OCH_2CH_3$. The "CH_3COCH_2" in the formula in the question cannot indicate an ether linkage because the second carbon atom will not have a full octet. (The carbon-oxygen bonds in an ether are single bonds.) Choice **C**, acid anhydride, has the general formula RCOOCOR'. Choice **D**, carboxylic acid, has the general formula RCOOH.

37. A
Constitutional isomers (also referred to as structural isomers) are isomers that differ in the connectivity of the atoms. The carbon skeletons may have completely different appearances, and the molecules may have different functional groups. For example, one may be an ether while the other may be an alcohol. For this question, we know from the molecular formula (which contains only C's and H's) that the isomers are all going to be hydrocarbons, so the task is to come up with the different possibilities for the carbon skeleton. Notice that the carbon-to-hydrogen ratio indicates that the compounds are all saturated, noncyclic hydrocarbons. (A noncyclic alkane has the general formula C_nH_{2n+2}. A formula of C_nH_{2n}, for example, would indicate either a noncyclic alkene with one double bond or a cyclic alkane.)

The best way to tackle the question is to write down the different possible structures for C_5H_{12}:

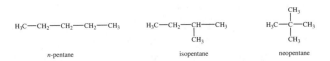

These three structures exhaust the possibilities for the formula C_5H_{12}. Any other structure that we can draw will turn out to be equivalent to one of these three possibilities, or will not be consistent with the formula. (Cyclopentane, for example, only has 10 hydrogen atoms.)

38. D
One of the things we are expected to do on the MCAT is to deduce something about the physical properties of a compound, especially relative to other analogous compounds. Physical properties refer to characteristics such as density, boiling point, melting point, solubility—properties that can be observed without having to subject the compound to any chemical reactions. Intermolecular attractions are a major factor in determining many physical properties, including boiling point. The stronger the attraction among the molecules, the higher the boiling point of the compound. Compounds capable of hydrogen bonding are generally expected to have higher boiling points than their non-hydrogen bonding counterparts, so carboxylic acids (choices **C** and **D**) are expected to have higher boiling points than ketones (choices **A** and **B**). In

fact, in the liquid state, carboxylic acid molecules form dimers held together by two hydrogen bonds instead of just one:

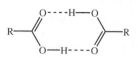

Within the same class of compounds, boiling point increases with molecular weight, since the compound with the higher molecular weight is generally larger and therefore engages in more dispersion interactions (another form of intermolecular attraction). Choice **D**, a carboxylic acid with eight carbon atoms, is therefore expected to have a higher boiling point than choice **C**, with seven carbon atoms.

39. D

Aromatic compounds are planar cyclic molecules with a conjugated pi system that is delocalized throughout the entire molecule. They are distinguished by a special amount of stability, as manifested in an unexpectedly low heat of hydrogenation for its pi bonds. (The first ones of these compounds studied happened to be fragrant, hence the term "aromatic." The term has stuck for purely historical reasons. Compounds considered aromatic in organic chemistry nowadays are no longer necessarily so.)

In addition to the planar and cyclic requirements mentioned above, an aromatic compound must also satisfy Huckel's rule by having a total of $(4n + 2)$ pi electrons, where n is some nonnegative integer. This requirement arose from molecular orbital considerations: The $(4n + 2)$ pi electrons reside in bonding rather than antibonding molecular orbitals.

Among the answer choices given, only choice **D** satisfies all the criteria. It is a planar cyclic molecule in which all the pi bonds are conjugated. (All the carbon atoms are sp^2-hybridized.) It has a total of seven pi bonds and hence 14 pi electrons. The molecule therefore satisfies Huckel's rule since $14 = 4 \times 3 + 2$; i.e., $n = 3$. It is an aromatic compound.

The compound in choice **A** is also cyclic and planar. With two pi electrons, it also satisfies Huckel's rule (with $n = 0$). However, these pi electrons are not delocalized. One of the carbon atoms is sp^3-hybridized and therefore does not have a p orbital through which the electrons can be delocalized:

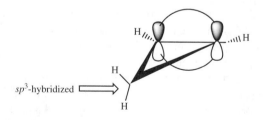

The compounds in choices **B** and **C** have four and eight pi electrons respectively, and neither number can be expressed in the form $(4n + 2)$, with n being a nonnegative integer. The compounds thus do not have the correct number of pi electrons to be aromatic.

40. D

A nitrogen atom with zero formal charge is basic by virtue of its lone pair of electrons, which can abstract a proton from an acid to form a quaternary ammonium salt. The more reactive the lone electron pair, the more basic the nitrogen atom. Conversely, the more stabilized the electron pair, the less basic the nitrogen atom. The nonbonding electron pair of each of the answer choices is shown explicitly below:

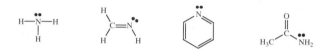

The amide in choice **D** has the least basic nitrogen atom, since the electron pair is resonance stabilized:

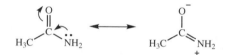

Because the electron pair is delocalized, it is not as "eager" to form a bond to a proton. The lone pair on ammonia (choice **A**) and on the imine (choice **B**) cannot be resonance stabilized. Nor can the electron pair in pyridine (choice **C**). The ring already has six pi electrons. The nonbonding electron pair resides in an sp^2-hybridized orbital that is in the same plane as the ring, so it is not delocalized.

41. C

The hydroxide ion is a strong nucleophile as well as a strong base, and dimethyl sulfoxide (DMSO) is a polar aprotic solvent. (An aprotic solvent is one that is incapable of participating in hydrogen bonds. Thus, water and alcohols are all protic solvents, but acetone and benzene are aprotic solvents.) The conditions are prime for a bimolecular reaction. The hydroxide ion attacks the alkyl halide, displacing the chloride group in a one-step (concerted) mechanism as follows:

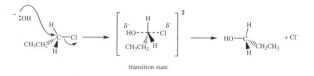

transition state

The reaction is an S_N2 reaction. It proceeds via a concerted mechanism: The attack of the hydroxide ion and the displacement of the leaving group occur in the same step, the one step that makes up the reaction. The rate law for a generic S_N2 reaction is rate = k[nucleophile][substrate]. In other words, the rate of the reaction is proportional to both the concentration of the nucleophile (in this case the hydroxide ion) and the concentration of the substrate (in this case 1-chloropropane). The statements in choices **B** and **D** are therefore both true and are not the correct answer.

Because the hydroxide ion is also a strong base, elimination (more specifically bimolecular elimination, E2) is a side reaction. The hydroxide ion acts as a base to abstract a proton from the carbon adjacent to the one bearing the halogen:

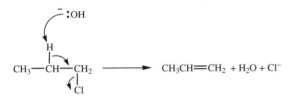

(The transition state is not shown.) An alkene is the product and the statement in choice **A** is therefore true.

The statement in choice **C** is false. Less substituted alkyl halides participate in S_N2 reactions more rapidly because the carbon to be attacked is more accessible. 1-Chloropropane is a primary alkyl halide: The carbon atom bearing the chlorine is bonded to only one alkyl group, making it relatively easy for the hydroxide ion to approach it. 2-Chloropropane, however, is a secondary alkyl halide. The halogen-bearing carbon is more sterically hindered because it is bonded to two alkyl groups. The hydroxide ion finds it harder to attack the carbon, making the reaction slower. We therefore find that the reactivity of alkyl halides in S_N2 reactions decreases as follows: methyl > primary > secondary > tertiary.

42. A

Molecular bromine will add across a carbon-carbon double bond to form a dibromo compound:

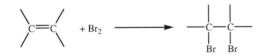

The reaction leads to a loss of the characteristic reddish-brown color of bromine, and is used as the basis for a qualitative test for the presence of unsaturation. However, the carbonyl bond of a ketone does not participate in this reaction, so choice **A** is the only correct answer.

The bromination of an alkene is an example of a large class of reactions known as addition reactions. In an addition

reaction, a double bond becomes saturated as sigma bonds to new groups are formed. Depending on the reaction conditions, the reaction can proceed through a variety of mechanisms and lead to many different types of products: alcohols, halohydrins, etc. The addition of a halogen (such as bromine), for example, proceeds via a cyclic intermediate:

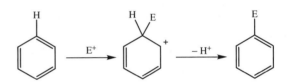

43. A

An electrophilic aromatic substitution (EAS) reaction is one in which an aryl hydrogen (a hydrogen directly attached to an aromatic ring) is replaced by another substituent. The reaction proceds through a carbocation intermediate:

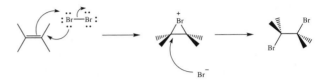

The substituent can be an alkyl group, a halogen, a nitro group, etc. (You should know the reagents used for different substituents for the MCAT.) The product can in principle undergo further substitution at another site either with the same or with a different electrophile. The rate of this further substitution is affected by the identity of the substituent already present on the ring. Substituents can be classified as activators or deactivators. Activators include (neutral) amine groups, the hydroxy group, alkoxy groups and alkyl groups. Their presence makes the compound more reactive (i.e., react more rapidly) in EAS reactions. Deactivators include halogens, the nitro group, the cyano group, and carbonyl groups. Their presence slows down the rate at which the compound reacts in EAS.

Choices **A** and **B** are both compounds with activating substituents. Methoxybenzene has the methoxy substituent $-OCH_3$, while toluene has the methyl group substituent. The methoxy group is more strongly activating than the methyl group, so the rate of EAS reaction will be most rapid for choice **A**.

44. B

The structure of 2-bromopropane is shown below. The molecule possesses two distinct proton types, labeled (a) and (b).

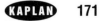

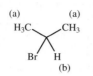

The protons from the two methyl groups are equivalent. There is therefore only one signal for the six protons. The signal is split by the proton labeled (b). The signal is therefore a doublet. Proton (b), in turn, is split by the six equivalent methyl protons. The signal is therefore a septet. For MCAT questions on NMR, it is important to master the concept of equivalent protons, and to be able to predict the splitting patterns that arise.

45. A

From an organic chemistry standpoint, one of the most interesting features of amino acids is their acid-base property. Every amino acid has a basic amino group and an acidic carboxyl group, as well as a side group that can potentially also be acidic or basic. An amino acid can therefore exist in several different protonation states depending on the pH of its environment. (An ability to interpret titration curves of amino acids is expected on the MCAT.)

In this question, the pH of the solution is higher than the pK value of every functionality of tyrosine, so each group acts as an acid towards the solvent. In other words, they all exist in the deprotonated, conjugate base form. The carboxyl group thus exists as the negatively charged carboxylate: $-COO^-$ instead of $-COOH$. The amino group exists as the neutral $-NH_2$ group instead of the $-NH_3^+$ group. The phenolic side chain exists as $-Ph-O^-$ instead of $-Ph-OH$. The structure of the amino acid at pH 11 is therefore as follows:

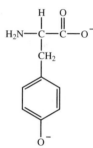

The net charge is therefore –2.

CHAPTER SEVEN

Biology

When confronted with an MCAT Biology passage, many students try to apply the same strategies they used during their undergraduate years: They try to read for understanding and focus on details mentioned in the passage. In doing so, they spend lots of time digesting the passage, which may result in running out of time before finishing the section. While reading for understanding and focusing on details may have worked for college courses, these strategies won't maximize your score on the MCAT. Since you have access to the passage at all times, you won't need to read for detail or understand everything about the passage to begin answering MCAT questions and earning points.

What can you do to manage your time most effectively and maximize your MCAT score? Read the passage only as needed and spend the majority of your time answering questions. Answering questions is what increases your score, not spending too much time reading passages.

READING THE PASSAGE

Passage Types

Information passages contain prose you might find in a textbook. They consist of paragraphs of text that are descriptive in nature. A passage may include a diagram or two related to the topic being discussed. For example, a typical information passage might discuss a particular disease, describe its symptoms, and include a pedigree illustrating its manner of inheritance. The majority of Biology passages on the MCAT are information passages.

Experiment passages describe one or more experiments and include a presentation of results. Since the results of the experiment or experiments are usually presented in table or graph form, these passages are often recognizable by the presence of tables and/or graphs. A diagram that illustrates an apparatus used in the experiment may also accompany the passage. For example, a typical experiment passage might present some background information about a topic, describe an experiment designed to investigate the topic, and use a table to present the results of the experiment.

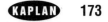

Persuasive argument passages consist mainly of paragraphs of text that explain one (or more) different viewpoints or hypotheses. For example, a typical persuasive argument passage might present background information about a disease, and present two hypotheses about the cause of the disease. Here is an example of a persuasive argument passage:

The human auditory system has the remarkable capacity to distinguish sound frequencies that differ by as little as 3 Hz, with a dynamic range of detection from 20 Hz to 20 kHz. The mechanism that provides this ability lies in the inner part of the ear, in an organ named the cochlea.

The cochlea is a fluid-filled tubular structure that is coiled into the shape of a seashell. Traversing the tube is a flat, rigid membrane known as the basilar membrane, upon which sit ciliated "hair cells" that are capable of transmitting an electrical signal through the auditory nerve back to the brain. A stiff gelatinous mass called the tectorial membrane overlies the hair cells.

A typical sound wave is conducted through the outer parts of the ear and induces minute vibrations at one end of the cochlea. These vibrations are then transmitted through the fluid inside and cause deflections in the basilar membrane proportional to the amplitude of the sound. Motion of the basilar membrane against the tectorial membrane causes the cilia on the hair cells to bend, mechanically triggering the opening of ion channels and causing the hair cells to "fire" like a neuron. Though this model accounts for the mechanism of sound detection, it does not explain how the frequency of a sound is encoded.

To date, two principles have been proposed governing the mechanism of sound frequency discrimination.

The Place Principle

The basilar membrane on which the hair cells sit vibrates differently along its length, with the base (the end facing the outer ear) the most sensitive to low frequency sounds, and the apex (the opposite end) most sensitive to high frequency sounds. According to the place principle, the brain can distinguish various frequencies based on the location of the hair cells that fire. Sounds of a specific frequency cause hair cells at a specific point along the basilar membrane to fire.

The Volley Principle

Neurons have the ability to fire in synchrony with a specific phase of a waveform, such that the frequency of neuronal firing will match the frequency of the sound vibration. This phenomenon is known as phase locking. According to the volley principle, sound frequency is simply encoded by the timing of the neuron's firing. Hence, a high frequency sound will cause a rapid rate of firing while a low frequency sound will lead to a slow rate of firing.

Remember that your goal is to get through a passage as quickly as possible so that you can spend the majority of your time answering questions. Answering questions is what earns you points on the MCAT. Be careful not to spend so much time digesting a passage that you run out of time when answering questions. As previously mentioned, MCAT passages contain a lot of information and data; however, it is important for you to remember that this information will always be there for you to refer to, should you need it. When reading a Biology passage, you should perform two tasks: *map the passage* and *identify the topic.*

MAPPING THE PASSAGE

The key to being able to access the information you need is creating a passage map. A passage map is a breakdown of the main ideas and critical concepts in a passage, paragraph by paragraph. By spending time reading for main ideas rather than details, and noting where concepts are presented in the passage, you'll spend less time reading a passage while still having enough of a grasp of the passage to know where to go for information should you need it to answer a question.

As you read a passage, determine what kind of passage it is. Depending on the type of passage, your strategy when reading the passage will be different. Use your knowledge of what makes up a particular passage type to help you. For example, does the passage consist of paragraphs of prose that are textbook-like and descriptive in nature? These are characteristics of information passages.

If the passage is an information passage, skim each paragraph and write down the main idea of each paragraph in the margin. As you read each paragraph, ask yourself, "What is the main idea of this paragraph?" You might find it easier to circle or underline the topic of each paragraph, but either way, the objective is to not get stuck trying to understand every detail of the passage, but to note the main ideas and go to the questions.

Does the passage contain a presentation of one or more experiments and a discussion of experimental design and results? Does the passage contain graphs and/or tables that present the results of an experiment? These are characteristics of experiment passages. Read experiment passages with the goal of understanding the what and the why of the experiment. If there are tables or graphs, note what quantities are being measured and any general trends.

Does the passage consist mainly of paragraphs of text that explain different viewpoints or hypotheses? Does the passage contain headings such as "Hypothesis I," "Hypothesis II," or "Scientist I," "Scientist II"? These are characteristics of persuasive argument passages.

In persuasive argument passages, read the paragraphs that explain the hypotheses or arguments carefully and try to grasp the main points of each of the hypotheses or arguments being presented. Note the main points of each hypothesis or argument in the margin, or underline the relevant sentences in each paragraph.

IDENTIFYING THE TOPIC

After reading the passage, note the topic of the passage. The topic of the passage is related to the type of passage. Recall from chapter 5 the following useful tips:

The topic of an information passage usually has the following format:

> *The passage describes/discusses* (phenomena).

The topic of an experiment passage usually has the following format:

> *The passage is about an experiment, the purpose of which is to* (purpose of experiment).

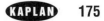

The topic of a persuasive argument passage usually has the following format:

The passage presents (<u>number</u>) *hypotheses about* (<u>phenomena</u>).

Here is a sample information passage, mapped using the strategies described in the previous section.

> Melanocytes are cells containing melanosomes, which are the cellular organelles responsible for synthesizing melanin. Melanin is a skin, hair, and retinal pigment synthesized from the amino acid tyrosine via an enzymatic reaction pathway.

Background information about melanocytes, melanin.

> Albinism is a genetic disorder in which melanin synthesis is blocked. In most forms of human albinism melanocytes appear to be normally distributed. Albinism occurs when a gene encoding an enzyme responsible for melanin production undergoes a mutation. As a result, individuals who suffer from albinism have extremely pale skin, white hair, and pinkish-colored eyes. They also experience vision problems because the eye's choroid, which is normally melanin-colored, is white. As a result, light entering the eye is reflected from, rather than absorbed into, the surface of the choroid and visual acuity is severely diminished. Albinos also run a greater risk for skin cancer, since the UV rays of the sun damage their unprotected skin cells.

Information about albinism: cause, symptoms.

> The frequency of the albino gene in the general population is 0.001, and is higher in many isolated populations, including the Amish and many Native American tribes. The pedigree in Figure 1 illustrates the pattern of inheritance for one form of human albinism.

Frequency of albino gene in general population and subpopulations

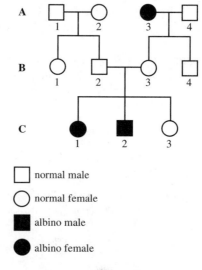

Figure 1

Pattern of inheritance of one form of human albinism.

Topic: The passage describes/discusses albinism.

Next is an example of an experiment passage; again, pay close attention to the mapping:

> Researchers discovered that cooking meat with charcoal results in the formation of polynuclear aromatic hydrocarbons on the food. To test whether these compounds are carcinogens, the Ames test is used. The Ames test identifies compounds that are chemical mutagens, and since most chemical mutagens are carcinogens, this test is able to ascertain carcinogenic risk.

Background information. The Ames test identifies chemical mutagens. Use of the Ames test to determine if polynuclear aromatic hydrocarbons are carcingens.

> In the Ames test, a mutant bacterial strain of *Salmonella typhimurium* unable to grow in the absence of histidine is placed on agar plates containing minimal growth media. (Minimal growth media lacks histidine.) A filter-paper disk with the suspected carcinogen and other compounds is placed in the center of the plates. The following four plates were used in this experiment.

Design of the experiment. A mutant bacterial strain is used that can't grow without histidine.

> Plate I: *Salmonella* alone
> Plate II: *Salmonella* + polynuclear aromatic hydrocarbons.
> Plate III: *Salmonella* + polynuclear aromatic hydrocarbons + human liver preparation
> Plate IV: *Salmonella* + 2-aminoanthracene (a known carcinogen).

Plate I: bacteria alone
Plate II: bacteria + test compound
Plate III: bacteria + test compound + human liver preparation
Plate IV: bacteria + known carcinogen

> The plates were incubated at 37°C for 48 hours. Only bacteria that regain the ability to synthesize histidine through *back-mutation* will be able to survive on these plates. The results of the experiments are shown in Figure 1.

More details about the experiment. Only bacteria that regain the ability to synthesize histidine will grow.

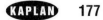

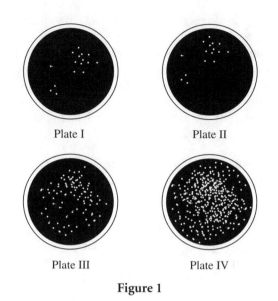

Figure 1

Results of the experiment. Plates I and II show little growth, while Plates III and IV show extensive growth. Plate IV shows the most growth.

Topic: The passage is about an experiment, the purpose of which is to determine whether polynuclear aromatic hydrocarbons are carcinogens.

Here is the sample persuasive argument passage presented earlier, mapped using the strategies described in the previous section.

> The human auditory system has the remarkable capacity to distinguish sound frequencies that differ by as little as 3 Hz, with a dynamic range of detection from 20 Hz to 20 kHz. The mechanism that provides this ability lies in the inner part of the ear, in an organ named the cochlea.

Background on the sense of hearing.

> The cochlea is a fluid-filled tubular structure that is coiled into the shape of a seashell. Traversing the tube is a flat, rigid membrane known as the basilar membrane, upon which sits ciliated "hair cells" that are capable of transmitting an electrical signal through the auditory nerve back to the brain. A stiff gelatinous mass called the tectorial membrane overlies the hair cells.

More background information.

> A typical sound wave is conducted through the outer parts of the ear and induces minute vibrations at one end of the cochlea. These vibrations are then transmitted through the fluid inside and cause deflections in the basilar membrane proportional to the amplitude of the sound. Motion of the basilar membrane against the tectorial membrane causes the cilia on the hair cells to bend, mechanically triggering the opening of ion channels and causing the hair cells to "fire" like a neuron. Though this model accounts for the mechanism of sound detection, it does not explain how the frequency of a sound is encoded.

How a sound wave is converted to an electrical signal to the brain.

> To date, two principles have been proposed governing the mechanism of sound frequency discrimination.

Two proposed principles regarding sound frequency discrimination.

> *The Place Principle*
>
> The basilar membrane on which the hair cells sit vibrates differently along its length, with the base (the end facing the outer ear) most sensitive to low frequency sounds, and the apex (the opposite end) most sensitive to high frequency sounds. Based on the place principle, the brain can distinguish various frequencies based on the location of the hair cells that fire. Sounds of a specific frequency cause hair cells at a specific point along the basilar membrane to fire.

The Place Principle: the location along the basilar membrane of the hair cells that fire encodes the frequency of the sound.

> *The Volley Principle*
>
> Neurons have the ability to fire in synchrony with a specific phase of a waveform, such that the frequency of neuronal firing will match the frequency of the sound vibration. This phenomenon is known as phase locking. According to the volley principle, sound frequency is simply encoded by the timing of the neuron's firing. Hence, a high frequency sound will cause a rapid rate of firing while a low frequency sound will lead to a slow rate of firing.

The Volley Principle: The timing of neuronal firing encodes the frequency of the sound.

Passage type: Persuasive argument

Topic: The passage presents two hypotheses about sound frequency discrimination.

HANDLING THE QUESTIONS

Recall the question types from chapter 5:

Discrete questions. These questions are not associated with any passage. They appear following a header such as "Questions 166–172 are NOT based on a descriptive passage." The Biological Sciences section contains 15 discrete questions spread throughout the section.

Here is an example of a discrete question:

> One form of hereditary diabetes is the result of an autoimmune disorder. The body produces antibodies that destroy its own insulin-producing cells. The most likely target of these antibodies are:
>
> **A.** pancreas cells.
> **B.** spleen cells.
> **C.** adrenal cells.
> **D.** liver cells.

Questions that require an understanding of the passage. These questions ask you to evaluate the validity of a hypothesis or argument given a new piece of information, determine what evidence would support a hypothesis or argument, or compare and contrast the hypotheses or arguments with each other. To answer these questions, you need to understand the concepts presented in the passage. Another example of a question that requires an understanding of the passage is the data interpretation/analysis question. These questions require you to interpret data from a table or graph, or analyze an experiment.

Here is an example of a question that requires an understanding of the passage:

Which of the following best accounts for the visible colonies on Plate I?

A.   Random mutations resulted in *Salmonella* cells that regained the ability to synthesize histidine.

B.   The cells were able to grow because histidine is not an essential amino acid for *Salmonella*.

C.   In the absence of one amino acid, *Salmonella* substituted a similar amino acid in its place.

D.   Foreign chromosome fragments containing the normal genes for histidine biosynthesis were transformed into a few *Salmonella* cells.

This question asks you to provide an explanation for the results of an experiment.

Questions where you need data from the passage. These questions can be answered without conceptual knowledge from the passage; however, you may need to go back to a specific part of the passage to retrieve data from a table, for example.

Here is an example of a question where you need data from the passage:

According to Figure 1, at what pO_2 are half the O_2-binding sites on Hb available?

A.   20 mm Hg

B.   25 mm Hg

C.   85 mm Hg

D.   90 mm Hg

You need to look at a graph to determine the answer to this question.

Questions that can stand alone from the passage. These questions can be answered without conceptual knowledge or data from the passage.

Here is an example of a question that can stand alone from the passage:

> Congenital defects in the skeletal structures of the limbs can be traced back to which of the following primary germ layer?
>
> A. Mesoderm
> B. Ectoderm
> C. Endoderm
> D. Notochord

This question can be answered without any information from the passage.

Certain question types appear more frequently with certain passage types. With an information passage, you will see more questions that can stand alone from the passage. With an experiment passage, you will see more questions where you need data from the passage. With persuasive argument passages, you will see more questions that require an understanding of the passage.

Handling the Questions

When answering Biology questions, be sure to go through the steps laid out in chapter 5:

Understand what you are being asked.

The first thing to do is read the entire question, including the answer choices. Reading the answer choices can help you focus your thoughts if the question stem by itself doesn't look particularly manageable. Using your reading comprehension skills, simplify the question to its bare essentials. Translate the question into your own words if necessary.

Here is a question that might appear with the passage about the experiment involving polynuclear aromatic hydrocarbons presented earlier:

> Which of the following best accounts for the visible colonies on Plate I?
>
> A. Random mutations resulted in *Salmonella* cells that regained the ability to synthesize histidine.
> B. The cells were able to grow because histidine is not an essential amino acid for *Salmonella*.
> C. In the absence of one amino acid, *Salmonella* substituted a similar amino acid in its place.
> D. Foreign chromosome fragments containing the normal genes for histidine biosynthesis were transformed into a few *Salmonella* cells.

Simplify/translate the question: what is it asking?

Here you are asked to provide an explanation for the results of an experiment.

Figure out where to go to get any information that you need.

Do you have enough information to answer the question? Do you need information from the passage?

> Which of the following best accounts for the visible colonies on Plate I?
>
> A. Random mutations resulted in Salmonella cells that regained the ability to synthesize histidine.
>
> B. The cells were able to grow because histidine is not an essential amino acid for Salmonella.
>
> C. In the absence of one amino acid, Salmonella substituted a similar amino acid in its place.
>
> D. Foreign chromosome fragments containing the normal genes for histidine biosynthesis were transformed into a few Salmonella cells.

This question asks for an explanation for the results of the experiment. Can you answer this question without referring to the passage? If you need information from the passage, refer to your passage map.

From your map of the passage, you should be able to quickly locate any information that you may need. Here, you are asked about the growth on Plate I. From our earlier discussion of question types, this is a question that requires an understanding of the passage. If you don't remember the results, look back at the passage to refresh your memory, using your passage map as a guide.

Here is a question that might appear with a passage about pattern formation:

> Congenital defects in the skeletal structures of the limbs can be traced back to which of the following primary germ layer?
>
> A. Mesoderm
>
> B. Ectoderm
>
> C. Endoderm
>
> D. Notochord

This question can be answered without any information from the passage.

Although this question might appear with a passage regarding pattern formation, you are not required to know any information from the passage. Even if you have not seen the passage, there is enough information given in the question stem to allow you to answer this question.

Integrating your science knowledge with any necessary passage research, determine the correct answer.

Which of the following best accounts for the visible colonies on Plate I?

A. Random mutations resulted in Salmonella cells that regained the ability to synthesize histidine.

B. The cells were able to grow because histidine is not an essential amino acid for Salmonella.

C. In the absence of one amino acid, Salmonella substituted a similar amino acid in its place.

D. Foreign chromosome fragments containing the normal genes for histidine biosynthesis were transformed into a few Salmonella cells.

This question asks for an explanation for the results of the experiment. Using your passage map, you referred to the diagram presenting the results of the experiment and noted that Plate I showed relatively little growth compared with Plates III and IV. Try to formulate an explanation before going through the answer choices. If you are stuck, go through all of the answer choices and use your reasoning skills to eliminate wrong answer choices.

This is the step where you bring together all the previous steps together with your science knowledge to determine the correct answer. Prior to arriving at this step, you need to understand what you are being asked and gather any information you may need from the passage. Once these tasks are accomplished, use your reasoning and/or calculation skills together with your science knowledge to arrive at the answer.

Try to formulate your own explanation before going through the answer choices. Plate I had *Salmonella* alone, with no other additional chemicals or preparations. In the absence of other factors, random mutations will cause some strains of *Salmonella* to acquire the ability to make histidine. Thus Choice **A** is the correct answer.

Alternatively, go through all of the answer choices. Choice **A** sounds reasonable, since random mutation brings about genetic variability in a population. Choice **B** is inconsistent with information presented in the passage. In Paragraph 2, it is stated that the *Salmonella* strain used in the experiment is unable to grow in the absence of histidine. This means that for this strain, histidine is an essential amino acid. Choice **C** does not make sense, since from the passage, this strain of *Salmonella* is unable to grow in the absence of histidine. Choice **D** is not possible, since the plate contains *Salmonella* alone, and no other organisms from which genetic material could be transformed into the *Salmonella*.

The next few pages contain a list of Biology concepts and skills you should have in your MCAT arsenal before Test Day.

IN PREPARING FOR THE MCAT, I SHOULD UNDERSTAND:

1. Molecular Biology

- Enzymes as biological catalysts
- Enzyme structure and function
- Competitive, noncompetitive, and feedback inhibition
- How enzymes are affected by changes in pH and temperature
- How a change in 3D structure affects an enzyme
- The difference between normal chromosomal inheritance and mitochondrial inheritance
- The basic structure of DNA and RNA
- How DNA is transcribed to RNA; regulation of transcription
- How RNA is translated to a polypeptide; regulation of transcription
- The structure and function of ribosomes
- Post-transcriptional modifications

2. Microbiology

- The basic structure of a bacterium
- Bacterial reproduction through binary fission
- How plasmids function in the transmission of bacterial genetic material
- The different processes by which bacteria can exchange genes: conjugation, transformation, and transduction
- The basic structure of a virus
- How bacteria and viruses differ
- The relative sizes of bacteria and viruses
- The general life cycle of a virus
- The mechanism of F plasmid transfer
- The characteristics of fungi: structural types, life history, and physiology

3. Generalized Eukaryotic Cell

- The functions of the major organelles
- The basic processes of cellular respiration and where they take place
- How the size of a typical eukaryotic cell compares to the size of a bacterium or virus
- Molarity and how a change in molarity affects a cell
- Structure and functions of the plasma membrane
- Osmosis, passive transport, active transport, endocytosis, exocytosis
- The structure and functions of the cytoskeleton
- Mitosis: where it falls in the cell cycle
- Mitosis: events that occur during each of the four phases
- The differences and similarities between mitosis and meiosis

 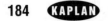

4. Specialized Eukaryotic Cells and Tissues

- The basic structure of nerve and muscle cells
- How nerve cells and muscle cells are specialized for their unique functions
- Membrane potential, resting potential, action potential
- Saltatory conduction
- How calcium functions in the regulation of muscle contraction
- The characteristics of different types of muscle: striated, smooth, and cardiac
- The characteristics of cartilage

5. Nervous and Endocrine Systems

- The organization of the nervous system
- The difference between sensor and effector neurons
- How a nervous impulse is transmitted across the synapse
- The sympathetic and parasympathetic nervous systems ("fight or flight" versus "rest and digest")
- The structure of the ear
- The mechanism of hearing
- The structure of the eye
- The mechanism of vision
- The mechanism of taste
- The mechanism of smell
- How steroid hormones utilize second messengers
- The major endocrine glands, what hormones they produce, what organs the hormones act on, and what their effects are
- Negative and positive feedback
- The cellular mechanisms of hormone action
- Hormone transport
- Homeostasis
- How pairs of hormones function in feedback loops to maintain homeostasis
- How a reflex arc works

6. Circulatory, Lymphatic, and Immune Systems

- The functions of the circulatory system
- The role of the circulatory system in thermoregulation
- The structure and function of the heart and blood vessels
- The path of blood flow through the body
- Systolic and diastolic blood pressure
- The composition of blood
- The characteristics of red blood cells that make RBCs ideal for transporting oxygen
- The major organs and structures of the immune system
- How the body develops tolerance to "self" antigens

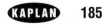

- The differences between the specific and nonspecific immune responses
- The roles of T- and B-lymphocytes in the immune response
- Where the cells of the immune system are produced and where they mature
- Antigens, antibodies, and antigen-antibody interaction
- The structures and functions of the lymphatic system

7.   Digestive and Excretory Systems

- The structures and functions of the digestive system
- Where each of the following is digested: protein, fat, carbohydrate
- What organs produce/store the various digestive enzymes, their substrates, and where they are secreted
- How the structure of the intestine enhances absorption of nutrients
- The structure and function of the kidney
- The structure and function of the nephron
- How urine is formed

8.   Muscle and Skeletal Systems

- What types of protein make up muscle fibers
- The functions of muscle
- The differences between voluntary and involuntary muscles
- How muscles contract, and the role of Ca^{++} and ATP
- The functions of the skeletal system
- The structure of bone
- The role of bone as a calcium reservoir
- The structure and function of joints
- The role of cartilage, ligaments, and tendons

9.   Respiratory and Skin Systems

- The structures of the respiratory system
- The mechanics underlying ventilation
- Where gas exchange takes place in the lung
- The role of surfactant in gas exchange
- The role of the respiratory system in thermoregulation, protection against disease, and protection against particulate matter
- The basic anatomy of the skin
- How the skin helps regulate temperature
- The role of the skin as an excretory organ
- The role of the skin as a protective barrier

10. Reproductive System and Development

- The structures and functions of the male and female reproductive tracts
- The processes of spermatogenesis and oogenesis (similarities and differences)
- The structure and functions of the placenta
- Embryogenesis: fertilization, cleavage, blastulation, gastrulation, neurulation
- The major structures derived from the three germ layers: ectoderm, mesoderm, endoderm
- The mechanisms of development: cell specialization; determination; differentiation; induction

11. Genetics and Evolution

- The advantages of sexual reproduction over asexual reproduction
- How to use a Punnett square to solve basic genetics problems
- Meiosis: where it falls in the cell cycle
- Meiosis: events that occur during each of the phases
- The differences and similarities between mitosis and meiosis
- How meiosis and random mutation increase the genetic variability in a population
- How the Kingdom/Phylum/Class/Order/Family/Genus/Species classification system works
- The concept of "fitness" in evolutionary terms
- The conditions for Hardy-Weinberg equilibrium
- How to apply the Hardy-Weinberg equations to population genetics problems

ng/mL of Tat from Exon 1 on nonactivated T-cells versus the effect of 1 ng/mL of Tat from Exon 1 on nonactivated T-cells. Looking at Table 1, you see that at either 1.25 micrograms or 2.5 micrograms of mRNA, there is *greater* TNF gene expression with 100 ng/mL of Tat than with 1 ng/mL of Tat. Therefore, it can be inferred that the *greater* the concentration of Tat from Exon 1 added to nonactivated cells, the *greater* the concentration of TNF mRNA. In other words, in nonactivated cells, the amount of TNF gene expression is *directly* proportional to the concentration of Tat from Exon 1.

To answer the question, find the most contrary, or opposite, trend. Since in nonactivated cells, the greater the Tat concentration the greater the TNF expression, you might have expected Tat to have the same effect on the activated cells of Cultures d_1 and d_2. However, if you look at the experimental results for the d cultures, the opposite occurs: In activated cells, the *greater* the Tat concentration the *less* TNF expression. In other words, there *is* greater repression of TNF gene expression at the *lower* concentration of Tat from Exon 1. This is contrary to the effect of the differing Tat concentrations on Cultures c_1 and c_2. Therefore, choice **A** is correct and choice **B** is incorrect. While choices **C** and **D** are true—there is greater TNF expression in the larger mRNA sample sizes and in Culture b than in Culture a—neither is unexpected in light of the effect of Tat concentration on nonactivated cells. So choice **C** and choice **D** are both incorrect.

35. B

In the question stem you're told that the Tat protein found circulating in the blood of an HIV-positive patient has a molecular weight less than half that of the peptide synthesized from the Tat gene inserted in a prokaryotic cell. Why the difference in molecular weight? The key to this is found in the first paragraph of the passage: The Tat protein is encoded by two exons spliced together. The only way to get two exons spliced together is if the RNA that linked them together was excised. You don't have to know the specifics of HIV genetics to answer this question, but here is some background information. The two exons that code for Tat are separated by a sequence of DNA that codes for other viral protein products. When Tat needs to be synthesized, *all* of this DNA is transcribed: The 2 Tat exons plus the DNA that links them. However, since the desired protein product is Tat, the RNA coding for the other proteins is excised and the two Tat exons are spliced together. All of this occurs within the nucleus of the eukaryotic host cell; remember, you're dealing with a retrovirus, which must integrate into the host genome before the viral genes can be expressed. Therefore, the initial mRNA transcript is longer than the transcript from which Tat is translated.

Prokaryotes do not perform post-transcriptional modification. The initial mRNA transcript is directly translated. Prokaryotes are *incapable* of such processing. Remember, in prokaryotes, there is no nucleus to separate transcription from translation. Therefore, if the viral DNA that contains the 2 Tat exons was inserted into a prokaryote, the mRNA transcribed and translated by the cell would consist of the codons coding for several viral proteins, not just Tat. This means that the protein synthesized from this mRNA transcript will be much longer and much heavier than the protein synthesized in the HIV-positive patient. Therefore, this prokaryotic protein couldn't rightfully be referred to as Tat.

Now examine the answer choices. The molecular weight of the protein would not be influenced by interaction with TNF—there's no information in the passage that would lead you to believe this; so choice **A** is incorrect. Choice **B** basically sums up the differences between eukaryotic and prokaryotic protein synthesis, and is the correct answer. Random mutations during synthesis could have caused the protein to have the same, a greater, or a smaller molecular weight depending on the nature of the mutation. However, because mutations are a *random* event, it is highly unlikely that all of the prokaryotic DNA would undergo mutations that resulted in a peptide twice the size of its eukaryotic counterpart. This is *not* the most likely explanation, and so choice **C** is not the answer. As for choice **D**, nowhere in the question stem does it say that the prokaryotic cells were exposed to PHA. Furthermore, exposure to PHA does not affect Tat weight or the weight of any proteins. Therefore, choice **D** is incorrect.

Discrete Questions (Questions 36–45)

36. A

The intermembrane space is the compartment between the outer and inner mitochondrial membranes. Protons are pumped from the matrix into the intermembrane space to create a proton motive force that is used to generate ATP during oxidative phosphorylation. Since the intermembrane space contains a high concentration of protons relative to the mitochondrial matrix (and cytoplasm), it will have an acidic pH. Only choice **A** contains a pH value in the acidic range (< 7).

37. A

To answer this question, you have to remember the function of the smooth endoplasmic reticulum (SER). The SER serves two major functions: Detoxification and lipid synthesis. Cholesterol and phospholipids are the main lipids synthesized.

Adrenal cortical cells would be expected to contain an abundant amount of SER because they synthesize steroid hormones (glucocorticoids and mineralocorticoids). Cholesterol is the building block of steroid hormones, and so adrenal cortical cells would require much SER in order to produce the corticoids necessary for homeostasis, answer choice **A**.

Epithelial cells and their cousins, endothelial cells, do not serve any capacity that involves the SER. These cells function primarily as a barrier. Adipose cells are the site of lipid storage, not synthesis. These cells also do not require an abundant amount of SER. An abundant amount of any organelle would take up precious storage space.

38. A
Statement I is a true statement since the two nucleotide strands of DNA are held together by hydrogen bonds (two bonds between thymine and adenine, three between guanine and cytosine).

Statement II is false because the phosphate groups that are part of the helical backbone are negatively charged. If anything, neighboring phosphate groups would repel one another, not attract.

Statement III is false because the sugar that is part of the DNA helix consists of deoxyribose, not ribose.

Since Statement I is true, and statements II and III are false, choice **A** is the correct answer.

39. D
If cells are removed from one location in an embryo and placed into another location, and they continue to develop as if they were not moved, the fate of the cells must have already been established. Such a cell is called *determined*, in which its developmental fate has been set even if the cell's appearance and function have not yet achieved their final state.

A totipotent cell, choice **A**, is a cell that has the capability to develop into any cell type of that organism. Only the very early cells of development, and the germ cells, are totipotent. Choice **B** is incorrect because the cells were not differentiated yet. A differentiated cell has completely matured into the cell type it will assume for the life of the organism. The cells in this experiment were removed while in the bud stage. The cells cannot be considered differentiated until they form an arm and all the associated structures. Choice **C** is incorrect because the cells developed normally, and so cannot be considered mutant. If a cell experiences damage to its genome that results in a phenotype that differs from normal, then it is mutant.

40. B
Directional selection produces an adaptive change over time in response to some change in the environment. When bacteria are exposed to antibacterial soaps, only those that are resistant will survive, leading to a prevalence of resistant genes in the bacterial gene pool. This is identical to the directional selection that occurs when insects become resistant to a pesticide.

Choice **A** is incorrect because a stabilizing selection maintains a uniform character by eliminating deviations. Choice **C** is incorrect because a disruptive selection favors extremes over the intermediate phenotypes. Choice **D** is incorrect because speciation is the evolution of a new species that can't interbreed with other species.

41. B
The question states that "osteoblasts secrete large quantities of alkaline phosphatase when they are actively depositing bone matrix." Thus, any condition that affects the activity of osteoblasts would affect the concentration of alkaline phosphatase in the circulation. Decreased dietary calcium intake would lead to a resorption of calcium from the bones. This is accomplished by osteoclasts, not osteoblasts. Therefore, there would be a decrease in osteoblast activity and a consequent decrease in alkaline phosphatase concentrations in the circulation.

Choice **C** is incorrect because osteoclasts exist within the bones and are not generally found in the circulation. Note that decreased dietary calcium also leads to increased osteoclast activity in order to maintain the concentration of Ca^{++} in the circulation. Choice **D** is incorrect because a decrease in dietary calcium tends to decrease $[Ca^{++}]_{plasma}$ and would be compensated for by increased resorption of calcium from the bones.

42. B
There are several ways to determine the mode of inheritance of a disease represented in a pedigree chart. The most thorough method would be to go through each of the answer choices and see if the mode of inheritance is possible by ascribing the appropriate genotypes to each of the individuals. Before resorting to that, use knowledge of genetics to eliminate answer choices. Below is a reproduction of the pedigree chart from the question, with each individual numbered and their genotypes listed.

First, notice in the P_1 generation that parents 1 and 2 do not have the disease, but some of their children do. Based on this, the disease cannot be dominant. If the disease were dominant, one or both of the parents must have the disease. You can therefore eliminate answer choices **A** and **C**. Next, notice that individual 7 is a female that has the disease, but her father does not. Based on this observation, the inheritance cannot be X-linked recessive. The steadfast rule is that for X-linked recessive traits, a female can express the trait only if her father expresses the trait. You can therefore eliminate choice **D**.

The above observations leave choice **B** as the correct answer.

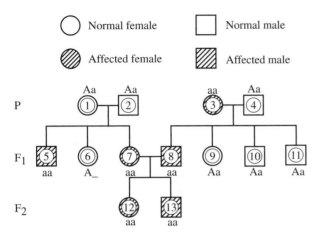

43. A

In meiosis I, the 46 chromosomes, each with two copies of the DNA, line up at the equator of the cell, and the paternal and maternal chromosomes segregate leaving two cells with 23 chromosomes each. These cells will then begin to undergo meiosis II. In meiosis II, the sister chromatids (copies of the same DNA) divide and four cells with 23 chromosomes (only one copy) are created.

For the MCAT, you should understand the processes of mitosis and meiosis, and also know the similarities and differences between the two processes. You should know in what types of body cells each type of division takes place (somatic versus germ cells), differences in the end products (diploid versus haploid), and the number of divisions that take place.

44. B

The nucleus of a zygote contains all the genetic information needed by all future cells of an adult organism in the form of genes. As the zygote divides and differentiates, each cell maintains *all* of its genetic information, but it does not *express* all of these genes; that is, certain genes are selectively expressed, while others are repressed. Gene expression is selectively turned on or off, depending on the type of cell. This is very important, because even though a myocardial cell may contain the same genetic information as an osteoblast, you wouldn't want to have your myocardial cells making bone in the middle of your heart. When certain genes that are normally turned *off* are mistakenly turned *on*, cancer can develop.

In this question, there is an experiment where the nucleus of a tadpole intestinal cell is removed and transplanted into a denucleated frog zygote. The zygote develops normally after the nucleus transplant. The experimental results suggest that a differentiated nucleus contains the same genetic material as a zygote's nondifferentiated nucleus. The fact that the nucleus was originally in a differentiated cell also suggests that selective repression of DNA is possible. This conclusion is fairly straightforward since, if the salvaged nucleus lacked genetic material essential to a developing tadpole, the zygote would develop into, at best, a mass of intestinal cells. If certain genes were missing, the zygote would not be able to develop normally. These conclusions about the experimental results are best represented by choice **B**.

Examine the wrong choices to make sure choice **B** is the best answer. Choice **A** says that the results of the experiment suggest that cell differentiation is controlled by irreversibly shutting off genes not needed by that cell. In fact, the experiment proves that this is *not* true and therefore choice **A** is incorrect. Shutting off genes must be reversible, otherwise this transplanted nucleus would *not* be able to direct the zygote to divide and develop into all of the different cell types found in a frog. Choice **C** suggests that the cytoplasm of the zygote contains all of the information needed for normal adult development in the form of RNA. This choice is incorrect because the experiment did *not* specifically address this question. The results of the experiment do not support or contradict this claim. Although DNA is the known carrier of genetic information, if you wanted to test the RNA theory, you would perform a different experiment, such as seeing if a denucleated frog zygote develops normally. As for choice **D**, all eukaryotic ribosomes are the same and are found only in the cytoplasm of a cell, not the nucleus. Again, choice **B** is the correct answer.

45. C

This question tests your understanding of red blood cells, the antigens they express on their cell surfaces, and the types of antibody production these antigens elicit. There are four major blood groups: A, B, AB, and O. There are three alleles determining these four groups: Alleles A and B are codominant, while allele O is recessive. The A allele codes for the A antigen on the red blood cell surface, the B allele codes for the B antigen, and the O allele does not code for any antigen. So, a person with type A blood has the genotype AA or AO, a person with type B blood is either BB or BO, a person with type AB blood has the genotype AB, and a person with type O blood is OO. A person's blood serum does not contain antibodies to any of its own antigens, but does contain antibodies to the other blood antigens. This means that a person with type A blood will have antibodies to the B antigen in their blood serum and a person with type B blood will have antibodies to the A antigen in their blood serum. A person with type AB blood would have neither anti-A nor anti-B antibodies since their red blood cells have both antigens. People with

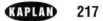

type O blood, on the other hand, will have both anti-A and anti-B antibodies since their red blood cells have neither the A nor B antigens.

The experiment in the question stem sets up four test tubes, numbered I through IV, with each test tube containing a different blood group. To each of these test tubes, type A red blood cells were added. To answer this question, you must determine which of these test tubes will form precipitate upon the addition of type A red blood cells. Precipitation occurs when the blood antigens react with their specific antibodies. Therefore, the test tubes containing blood serum with anti-A antibodies will form precipitate. The two blood types that will produce anti-A antibodies are type B and type O blood. Therefore, precipitate will form in test tube II, which contains type B blood, and test tube IV, which contains type O blood. Precipitate will not form in the other blood types because they do not contain the anti-A antibody. So the correct answer is choice **C**.

section III

VERBAL REASONING AND WRITING SAMPLE

CHAPTER EIGHT

Verbal Reasoning

The Verbal Reasoning section is perhaps the most familiar section of the MCAT, since it's similar to the reading comprehension sections of other standardized tests. The section is 85 minutes long and usually consists of 9 passages, with 6–10 questions per passage for a total of 65 multiple-choice questions. (Beginning in 2003, the section will go down to 60 questions in 85 minutes.) The passages are drawn from those natural sciences not included in the science portions of the test, and from the social sciences and humanities.

The science portions of the MCAT test your ability to work with the kind of information in which you have, or are expected to develop, expertise. The verbal sections test your reasoning abilities in working with material in which you are *not* expected to develop expertise.

The AAMC Verbal Reasoning question categories are:

Comprehension
- Global: main idea, author's purpose
- Details: answers stated expressly in the passage
- Deduction: inferences and assumptions

Evaluation
- Identify the function of a statement
- Describe the structure of the passage

Application
- Apply ideas in the passage to new information

Incorporation
- Apply new information to arguments made in the passage

WHAT SKILLS ARE REWARDED IN VR?

- The ability to stay "on point," that is, to concentrate and not get distracted
- The ability to switch gears quickly from one passage and topic to the next
- The ability to recognize the overall purpose of a paragraph
- The ability to process large and small pieces of data and find a pattern within them
- Stamina

All of these have considerable applicability to medical school and your career as a physician.

DO YOU NEED TO PREPARE FOR VERBAL REASONING?

Don't make the mistake of underestimating the challenge of the Verbal Reasoning section. The scoring gradient for Verbal Reasoning is very steep, and some medical schools add all your MCAT scores together for a composite score, so you can't afford to be cavalier.

We generally read for entertainment or information. MCAT Verbal Reasoning requires that you abandon standard reading habits and take on the role of a critical reader. To concentrate and glean meaning regardless of the nature of the text will mean working through your resistance to dry passages and overcoming anxiety or frustration. The more control you can muster, the quicker you can move through each passage, through the questions, and to a higher score.

ESTABLISH AND ADHERE TO A SCHEDULE

If you're serious about improving your performance on MCAT VR, start now to establish and follow a practice schedule. VR requires that you internalize methods and strategies; there's nothing here that you can memorize at the last minute.

Rough Calendar

Set up a timetable that works for you. Be realistic but demanding of yourself.

Set up a blank calendar for the period between now and Test Day, broken down by months/weeks, or weeks/days, depending on how much time is left. Insert upcoming holidays (and allow yourself some time off). Then develop and build a proper study schedule. Here are some general principles:

- Assess the practice material available from AAMC and schedule that practice to develop your skills early and keep them strong.
- Keep working on small groups of passages until the day before your Test Day.
- Don't work on Verbal Reasoning for more than 120–150 minutes at a time.

On Test Day itself, plan to warm up your Verbal Reasoning skills with an old passage or two and its questions. To get off to a positive start, if this section is a problem for you, find an inviting passage and get it done first!

 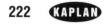

Practice Tests and Passages

Time yourself on practice sets and tests, allowing 27 minutes for 3 passages (rather than timing each passage). Practice can establish a sense of pacing that will become second nature by Test Day.

Practice at the same time of day that you'll be starting on Test Day, since Verbal Reasoning is the first section.

Three things to be careful of:

- Don't be discouraged by the errors you make. Errors made in practice give you the opportunity to identify your strengths and weaknesses and focus on modifying your habits.
- Don't wait too long to review explanations after taking a practice test.
- Don't do more than two passages at a time without taking a break; sensory overload will cause you to lose focus.

Outside Reading

Select materials of the kinds that will appear in VR but that you don't normally read. Take on at least one difficult outside-reading challenge per week. Sources of such outside reading include: *The Economist, Archaeology, Scientific American, The New York Times* Op-Ed pages, *Atlantic Monthly, Foreign Affairs, Modern Art, The New York Review of Books*—and see what literary and professional journals are available at your local library.

If possible, make two photocopies of the articles, one with the title and source hidden. Keep a log of your outside reading, and check it from time to time to ensure that you're keeping to your schedule and reading a good variety of disciplines. By continuing to read and analyze difficult pieces of prose you ensure that all of your skills will be sharp on Test Day.

Don't just read, critically read. One purpose of your outside reading is to increase your comfort and familiarity with the kinds of writing you'll find on the test, but the other is to practice all the Kaplan methods and strategies. Do these things as you practice critical reading:

- Practice mapping paragraphs (as we'll discuss below).
- Ask yourself the author's purpose.
- Think about the standard VR question types that can be asked based on material you've read.
- Notice your comfort levels and reading pace, and plan further reading to overcome problem areas.

THE KAPLAN METHOD FOR VERBAL REASONING

The Kaplan Method for Verbal Reasoning is:

Step 1: Select a Passage

Step 2: Critically Read the Passage

Step 3: Interpret the Question Stem

Step 4: Review Your Map and Text

Step 5: Make a Prediction

Step 6: Read the Choices

We'll discuss each step briefly first, then examine them in more detail with some of the strategies incorporated.

Step 1: Select a Passage

When you find a passage difficult, skip it until you've finished the others. One question is not worth more than another; don't let a difficult passage keep you from getting to easier passages and questions. But this doesn't mean wasting precious minutes looking at all the passages before you decide which you'll do first, second, or third. Look at the first passage on your test and, if it isn't a type that gives you special trouble, start to read it. As long as you're not too far into the passage, skip to the next one if, for any reason, a passage you've begun to read slows you down seriously. But keep in mind that:

- You are going to read all of the passages and answer all of the questions—your triage affects only the order in which you do them.
- Many students find that they make more mistakes with passages on topics they are familiar with than on topics they don't like (because of their tendency to rely on outside knowledge rather than the passage).
- The questions in Verbal Reasoning tend to get harder as you progress through the section—so skipping early passages means skipping easy questions!

Step 2: Critically Read the Passage

Reading and mapping Verbal Reasoning passages is different in important ways from the process used on science passages, principally because outside knowledge is irrelevant here, and the content is less important than the structure. To read passages critically means:

- Using Keywords to help you navigate the passage
- Capturing the gist by paraphrasing
- Identifying the topic, scope, and purpose of the passage
- Creating a map of the passage structure to locate details as required

The most important statements in any Verbal Reasoning passage are those in which conclusions (which we'll also call "opinions") are expressed. A passage may consist only of the author's opinion, or you may find two or more contrasted opinions. Sentences in which the *author's voice* is heard clue you in to the *author's purpose* in writing the passage. *Opinion sentences* shed light on the direction in which the text is moving—they provide a map that you can use to organize your thoughts about the text. And they direct your pacing—you should read opinions more carefully than supporting detail, and paraphrase them when you're done.

 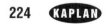

Step 3: Interpret the Question Stem

Read the question stem to answer two questions:

First: Exactly what does the question ask?

Pay close attention: If you misread the question, all your other work will be wasted. Many standard "wrong answer choices" are based on common misreadings of the question (for example, they can be the opposite of what is asked). *Annotate* the question stem. Some words (such as LEAST, EXCEPT, NOT, *strengthen*, or *weaken*) are "preannotated" for you, but you should highlight other essential terms that will help you find the answer. Many mistakes are made by losing sight of an essential element of the question.

Second: Do you expect to find the answer explicitly stated in the passage?

The stem may direct you to relevant text by line or paragraph number, or by direct quotes from the passage; or it may use names or other words that appear (sometimes repeatedly) in the text without any indication that they are quoted.

Step 4: Review Your Map and Relevant Text

With the details of the question in mind, reground yourself in the passage—use the Map you created by paraphrasing and annotating the passage to locate any relevant text. This step is easiest when the question refers to lines of text, a particular paragraph, or a specific argument. But some regrounding in the passage is helpful for every question type, even if it's only a review of the broad outlines of the passage and the author's scope and purpose. Even when you believe you remember the exact words in the passage that answer the question, you may find that you've overlooked a relevant detail.

Step 5: Make a Prediction

Before you consult the answer choices, predict the content, or at least the broad outline, of the correct answer. Most often, this will require argument dissection skills that we'll discuss in detail below. Predicting your answer will speed up and focus your search among the choices and reduce your chances of being misled by a plausible wrong answer.

Step 6: Read the Choices

Armed with your predictions and refreshed on the relevant text, you'll be ready to look for the right choice. Pay close attention to the wording of the answer choices—only one will be valid based on the passage. Read all the choices before selecting one—sometimes a wrong answer choice varies from the correct choice very subtly.

Before we start our in-depth analysis of the Kaplan strategies, let's try a practice passage with one of each of the AAMC question types. Critically read the passage below. Consider what the author is trying to say and how the ideas are communicated. Pause after each paragraph to paraphrase its ideas. On the following page are six questions; don't spend more than five or six minutes answering them.

Revisionist historians maintain that it was within the power of the United States, in the years during and immediately after the Second World War, to prevent the Cold War with the Soviet Union. Revisionists
5 suggest that the prospect of impending conflict with the Soviets could have been avoided in several ways. The U.S. could have officially recognized the new Soviet sphere of influence in Eastern Europe instead of continuing to call for self-determination in those
10 countries. A much-needed reconstruction loan could have helped the Soviets recover from the war. The Americans could have sought to assuage Soviet fears by giving up the U.S. monopoly of the atomic bomb and turning the weapons over to an international
15 agency (with the stipulation that future nuclear powers do the same).

This criticism of the post-war American course of action fails to take into account the political realities in America at the time, and unfairly condemns the
20 American policy-makers who did consider each of these alternatives and found them to be unworkable. Recognition of a Soviet Eastern Europe was out of the question. Roosevelt had promised self-determination to the Eastern European countries, and the American
25 people, having come to expect this, were furious when Stalin began to shape his spheres of influence in the region. The President was in particular acutely conscious of the millions of Polish-Americans who would be voting in the upcoming election.

30 Negotiations had indeed been conducted by the administration with the Soviets about a reconstruction loan, but the Congress refused to approve it unless the Soviets made enormous concessions tantamount to restructuring their system
35 and withdrawing from Eastern Europe. This, of course, made Soviet rejection of the loan a foregone conclusion. As for giving up the bomb—the elected officials in Washington would have been in deep trouble with their constituents had that plan been
40 carried out. Polls showed that 82 percent of the American people understood that other nations would develop bombs eventually, but that 85 percent thought that the U.S. should retain exclusive possession of the weapon. Policy-makers have to abide
45 by certain constraints in deciding what is acceptable and what is not. They, and not historians, are in the best position to perceive those constraints and make the decisions.

Revisionist historians tend to eschew this type of
50 political explanation of America's supposed failure to reach a peaceful settlement with the Soviets in favor of an economic reading of events. They point to the fact that in the early post-war years American businessmen and government officials cooperated to expand
55 American foreign trade vigorously and to exploit investment opportunities in many foreign countries. In order to sustain the lucrative expansion, revisionists assert, American policy-makers were obliged to maintain an "Open Door" foreign policy, the object of
60 which was to keep all potential trade opportunities open. Since the Soviets could jeopardize such opportunities in Eastern Europe and elsewhere, they had to be opposed. Hence, the Cold War. But if American policy-makers were simply pawns in an
65 economic game of expansionist capitalism, as the revisionists seem to think, why do the revisionists hold them responsible for not attempting to reach an accord with the Soviets? The policy-makers, swept up by a tidal wave of capitalism, clearly had little control
70 and little choice in the matter.

Even if American officials had been free and willing to make conciliatory gestures toward the Soviets, the Cold War would not have been prevented. Overtures of friendship would not have been
75 reciprocated (as far as we can judge; information on the inner workings of the Kremlin during that time is scanty). Soviet expert George F. Kennan concluded that Russian hostility could not be dampened by any effort on the part of the United States. The political
80 and ideological differences were too great, and the Soviets had too long a history of distrust of foreigners—exacerbated at the time by Stalin's rampant paranoia, which infected his government— to embark on a process of establishing trust and peace
85 with the United States, though it was in their interest to do so.

1. The primary purpose of the passage is to:

   A. criticize historical figures.

   B. refute an argument.

   C. analyze an era.

   D. reconcile opposing views.

2. The author refers to the Polish-Americans chiefly to illustrate that:

   A. the president had an excellent rapport with ethnic minorities.

   B. immigrants had fled from Eastern European countries to escape communism.

   C. giving up the idea of East European self-determination would have been costly in political terms.

   D. the Poles could enjoy self-determination only in America.

3. A fundamental assumption underlying the author's argument in the third and fourth paragraphs is that:

   A. the American public was very well-informed about the incipient Cold War situation.

   B. none of the proposed alternatives would have had its intended effect.

   C. the American public was overwhelmingly opposed to seeking peace with the Soviets.

   D. the government could not have been expected to ignore public opinion.

4. The author would consider which of the following an example of the "certain constraints" (line 45) that policy-makers are subject to?

   A. the etiquette of international diplomacy

   B. the danger of leaked information about atomic bombs

   C. the views of the electorate

   D. the potential reaction of the enemy

5. Which statement best summarizes the revisionist argument concerning the origin of the Cold War?

   A. The Soviets were oblivious to the negative impact they had on the American economy.

   B. The economic advantage of recognizing Soviet Europe outweighed the disadvantage of an angry public.

   C. America could trade and invest with foreign countries only if it agreed to oppose the Soviet Union.

   D. American economic interests abroad would have been threatened by any Soviet expansion.

6. Which of the following, based on the information in the passage, would most strengthen the author's judgment about the likelihood that the Cold War could have been averted?

   A. evidence that the author has no anti-communist bias

   B. new documents giving a complete picture of the hostility of the Soviets to American conciliatory gestures

   C. support for the author's views by a noted authority

   D. a demonstration of alternatives not suggested by the Revisionists

Turn the page to read an example of what the passage looks like when mapped. How do your thoughts match the notes that follow the paragraphs? Following the passage map are the answers and explanations for the six questions. For each question you got right, could you have answered it more quickly? For each question you missed, why did you get it wrong? What can you fix about your approach to VR questions so that you won't make the same mistake again?

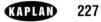

MAPPING THE PASSAGE

Revisionist historians <u>maintain</u> that it was within the power of the United States, in the years during and immediately after the Second World War, to prevent the Cold War with the Soviet Union. Revisionists <u>suggest</u> that the prospect of impending conflict with the Soviets could have been avoided in <u>several ways</u>. The U.S. could have officially recognized the new Soviet sphere of influence in Eastern Europe instead of continuing to call for self-determination in those countries. A much needed reconstruction loan could have helped the Soviets recover from the war. The Americans could have sought to assuage Soviet fears by giving up the U.S. monopoly of the atomic bomb and turning the weapons over to an international agency (with the stipulation that future nuclear powers do the same).

This criticism of the post-war American course of action <u>fails</u> to take into account the political realities in America at the time, and <u>unfairly condemns</u> the American policy-makers who did consider each of these alternatives and found them to be unworkable. Recognition of a Soviet Eastern Europe was out of the question. Roosevelt had promised self-determination to the Eastern European countries, and the American people, having come to expect this, were <u>furious</u> when Stalin began to shape his spheres of influence in the region. The President was in particular acutely conscious of the millions of Polish-Americans who would be voting in the upcoming election.

Negotiations had indeed been conducted by the administration with the Soviets about a reconstruction loan, <u>but</u> the Congress <u>refused</u> to approve it unless the Soviets made <u>enormous concessions</u> tantamount to restructuring their system and withdrawing from Eastern Europe. This, of course, made Soviet rejection of the loan a foregone conclusion. As for giving up the bomb—the elected officials in Washington would have been in <u>deep trouble</u> with their constituents had that plan been carried out. Polls showed that 82 percent of the American people understood that other nations would develop bombs eventually, but that 85 percent thought that the U.S. should retain exclusive possession of the weapon. Policy-makers have to abide by certain constraints in deciding what is acceptable and what is not. They, and not historians, are in the <u>best position</u> to perceive those constraints and make the decisions.

Paragraph 1 explains the three things that, according to the Revisionists, could have been done to avoid the Cold War.

One way

Second way

Third way

Topic/Scope: the Cold War, and why Revisionists are wrong

The author refutes these arguments; the American political atmosphere made these steps impossible.

Response to argument #1 above

Note strong judgmental and emotional words—it isn't necessary to catch, let alone annotate, each of them, but pick up on how they structure the argument.

Response to #2

Response to #3

More of the author's judgment

Revisionist historians tend to eschew this type of political explanation of America's supposed failure to reach a peaceful settlement with the Soviets in favor of an economic reading of events. They point to the fact that in the early post-war years American businessmen and government officials cooperated to expand American foreign trade vigorously and to exploit investment opportunities in many foreign countries. In order to sustain the lucrative expansion, revisionists assert, American policy-makers were obliged to maintain an "Open Door" foreign policy, the object of which was to keep all potential trade opportunities open. Since the Soviets could jeopardize such opportunities in Eastern Europe and elsewhere, they had to be opposed. Hence, the Cold War. But if American policy-makers were simply pawns in an economic game of expansionist capitalism, as the revisionists seem to think, why do the revisionists hold them responsible for not attempting to reach an accord with the Soviets? The policy-makers, swept up by a tidal wave of capitalism, clearly had little control and little choice in the matter.

Even if American officials had been free and willing to make conciliatory gestures toward the Soviets, the Cold War would not have been prevented. Overtures of friendship would not have been reciprocated (as far as we can judge; information on the inner workings of the Kremlin during that time is scanty). Soviet expert George F. Kennan concluded that Russian hostility could not be dampened by any effort on the part of the United States. The political and ideological differences were too great, and the Soviets had too long a history of distrust of foreigners—exacerbated at the time by Stalin's rampant paranoia, which infected his government—to embark on a process of establishing trust and peace with the United States, though it was in their interest to do so.

Revisionists would claim the economic situation forced policy-makers to oppose the Soviets.

If American officials were caught in an economic tide why blame them for not doing things differently?

There was no way the Cold War could have been avoided. Soviets were hostile, paranoid—a new argument.

The author of this passage has one overarching strategy and carries it out in a classic VR passage structure: Set up the arguments of the Revisionist historians and then refute that position throughout the rest of the passage. When a VR passage begins with a "traditional" view, or a statement of what others believe, expect to see the author's subsequent opposition.

1. B

When answer choices all start with verbs (as they frequently do in "purpose" and "main idea" questions), a vertical scan of the verbs can quickly reduce the number of answer choices you have to read in full. As we noted above, the author of this passage is primarily engaged in setting up and knocking down the arguments of the Revisionists. This makes **B** correct and **D** wrong (the author is definitely not interested in reconciling his view with that of the Revisionists.) **A** is out because the author is defending historical figures—the policymakers—for what they did, not criticizing them. **C** is too neutral a choice for this passage; the author does engage in analysis of the era of the beginning of the Cold War, but his purpose is to do far more than just analyze events—he wants to rebut the Revisionist theories. "Main idea" questions are rare on MCAT VR, but knowing the main idea is helpful in answering Deduction questions and in eliminating wrong answer choices.

2. C

For this Evaluation question, look at the second half of paragraph 2, where the author says Roosevelt could never have recognized a Soviet Eastern Europe because the American people did not like the idea of the Soviets holding sway in that region. In particular, the president would have lost the votes of the Polish-Americans who, you can infer, did not want the Soviets controlling their "old country." **C** spells out this point. Each of the other choices misreads the sentence about the Polish-American voters.

3. D

Deduction questions are the most common in VR sections. To identify an assumption, identify the evidence and conclusion, and find the connection between them. In the second and third paragraphs, the author refutes the suggestions of the revisionists primarily by saying that the policy-makers couldn't do what was necessary to avoid the Cold War because the American people were against it. The assumption the author makes is that the policy-makers "could not have been expected to ignore public opinion," as stated in answer choice **D**. The author never says in the second and third paragraphs that none of the alternatives would work (**B**)—what he does say, in a later paragraph, is that if peace initiatives had not run aground due to American politics, then they would have run aground due to the Soviet climate. The author also does not say in the second and third paragraphs that the American public was "well-informed" (**A**) or "overwhelmingly opposed to seeking peace" (**C**); all we know is that they opposed Soviet influence in Eastern Europe as well as the idea of giving up the atom bomb monopoly.

4. C

This Application question is closely linked to the previous one. This is a common phenomenon in VR, so if a question is difficult, answer the other questions for the passage before coming back to it. Here, the author refers to the "certain constraints" at the end of the third paragraph, in the midst of the discussion on the impact of public opinion on the policy-makers. From context, then, you know that the constraints the author is talking about are the opinions of the people—in other words, "the views of the electorate," answer choice **C**. If you didn't put the sentence about "constraints" in context, any of the other choices might have looked appealing.

5. D

This is a Detail question, merely asking that you paraphrase something stated in the passage. This question centers on paragraph 4, where the author explains the Revisionists' view that American policy-makers decided to oppose the Soviet Union because Soviet expansion could jeopardize United States trade and investment. Answer choice **D** captures this idea. The author says nothing about whether or not the Soviets knew about the negative impact they could have on the American economy, as stated in answer choice **A**. Choice **B** is out because the Soviet Union was not recognized by the United States, so this could not possibly have had anything to do with the origin of the Cold War. **C** is wrong because there is no evidence in the paragraph to support it.

6. B

Finally, an Incorporation question. The author's judgment is that the Revisionists are wrong: The Cold War could not have been averted due to American attitudes and Russian hostility. He does admit, however, that there isn't much information about what was going on in the Kremlin at the time, so he can't be totally sure of the latter argument. B is therefore the correct answer. This argument would not be affected by evidence of the author's feelings against communism (answer choice **A**), or the contrary opinion of a "noted authority" (**C**), or the viability of other alternatives (**D**).

SELF-EVALUATION

For students hoping only to "pass" a test, simply taking many practice tests will probably improve their score. But if you're already performing well and want to improve, constant self-evaluation is key. Make this a regular part of your preparation for Verbal Reasoning.

Instead of reviewing the explanations to questions completely, many students stop at seeing why one answer is correct. This is a costly mistake if you want to maximize your score. Learn all you can about your strengths and weaknesses between now and Test Day, then use that information to manage your test taking. Some people find they make certain mistakes consistently; others only find some tendency toward certain errors. In either case, you can reduce, or even eliminate, the problem if you recognize it.

After taking practice Verbal Reasoning test sections, fill in a copy of the Self-Evaluation form at the end of this subsection for all 35 questions. Then check which answers you got right. This will help you to identify any question type that you need to review and practice more, and give you a better sense of when you can trust your instincts on questions you're unsure of.

After practice sets or tests, consider the following questions:

Order of Attack: Are you comfortable, in retrospect, with the order in which you tackled the passages? What decisions do you regret? Satisfy yourself that you are taking control of the section, skipping difficult passages until you complete more manageable ones.

Time Management: Did you spend too much time on any passage?

Kaplan Methods and Strategies: Did you use Kaplan's methods and strategies in the course of this practice session? These should be practiced until they're second nature.

Fatigue: Did you start to make more mistakes later in the test? If so, you have to build your stamina methodically. Consider, too, taking minibreaks. Periodically put down your pencil, close your eyes and take deep breaths for 15–30 seconds, then go back to work.

Why did you get questions wrong? Get away from the sheer fact of getting a question wrong to learning to reconstruct where and how. The most common reasons for going wrong are:

> *Misreading the passage:* That is, misunderstood what the passage was saying, or went to the wrong part of the passage.
>
> *Misreading the question:* Questions that are easy to misread are reasoning questions, or the questions that employ the words LEAST/EXCEPT/NOT—perhaps you'll find you have a tendency to misread other types. Check the question one last time before settling on a final answer.
>
> *Misreading the choices:* Quite common.
>
> *Mismanaging time:* Ran out of time and became too pressed.

Why did you REJECT the right answer? When you pick a wrong answer, you reject the right one. Can you see any pattern in what you thought was wrong with the answer that turned out to be the correct one? Often the answer to this is one of the following:

> *Nit-picked it.* Some students object to a preposition or adverb in the credited choice, rather than taking the choice in its totality. Don't fight the test. The right answers are rarely perfect.

Misread it. Hasty test takers are prey to this error. The best defense here is, of course, to read each choice as it's worded.

Never read it. Students often (out of panic usually) go with the first choice that looked good. This is a bad habit based on false economy.

Some Self-Evaluation Experiments

Looking Ahead at the Questions

Some test takers feel more anchored as they read the passage if they've glanced at the questions first. As a rule, it won't save you time or effort to do so. Most of the questions require a general understanding of the passage. You need to read for meaning and for organization whether or not you've reviewed the questions. However, you may find that a very quick look to identify the subjects of the questions (and any line or paragraph references) helps you to focus on those areas as you read. Experiment with the possible benefits of looking at the questions before you read, and use this technique if it works for you.

One caveat, though. If you decide you can benefit from a preview of the questions, *don't look at the choices.* Some of you may know that the official test maker word for wrong answers is "distractors"—they're designed to confuse and mislead, and you don't want information from the choices clouding your comprehension of the passage.

Reading Speed

Finding your ideal reading pace is essential to maximizing your score in VR. To do this, try reading a few passages differently. If you believe you tend to get bogged down in passages, try practicing the fastest skimming you can do and still glean the broad outline—the structure. If you believe you tend to skim too quickly, try forcing yourself to slow down; actually read each sentence and paraphrase each paragraph.

Then do the questions and see how your results compare with your usual reading speed. If you do about as well with the radically different speed, your best speed lies midway between the two. If you do significantly better at one extreme than at the other, your best speed lies closer to the former speed.

Annotation Style

By Test Day, you should have developed an annotation style that works well for you. For some students, that means copious notes and a diversity of markings in the passage, while others find that the less they note the better. Your goal is to make as little notation as possible while still establishing and retaining a strong sense of the passage structure. Start with full paraphrases of the ideas in each passage and regular annotation—then strip your paraphrases and annotations down until you find a point at which your ability to respond to questions starts to drop—and return to the next higher level of "mapping."

The next couple of pages contain the self-evaluation form. Photocopy it and use it as often as possible as you work with full-length Verbal sections from AAMC *Practice Tests I–VI*.

SELF-EVALUATION FORM

1. GL DT DD EV AP IN
   vs ps us gu   Right Wrong

2. GL DT DD EV AP IN
   vs ps us gu   Right Wrong

3. GL DT DD EV AP IN
   vs ps us gu   Right Wrong

4. GL DT DD EV AP IN
   vs ps us gu   Right Wrong

5. GL DT DD EV AP IN
   vs ps us gu   Right Wrong

6. GL DT DD EV AP IN
   vs ps us gu   Right Wrong

7. GL DT DD EV AP IN
   vs ps us gu   Right Wrong

8. GL DT DD EV AP IN
   vs ps us gu   Right Wrong

9. GL DT DD EV AP IN
   vs ps us gu   Right Wrong

10. GL DT DD EV AP IN
    vs ps us gu   Right Wrong

11. GL DT DD EV AP IN
    vs ps us gu   Right Wrong

12. GL DT DD EV AP IN
    vs ps us gu   Right Wrong

13. GL DT DD EV AP IN
    vs ps us gu   Right Wrong

14. GL DT DD EV AP IN
    vs ps us gu   Right Wrong

15. GL DT DD EV AP IN
    vs ps us gu   Right Wrong

16. GL DT DD EV AP IN
    vs ps us gu   Right Wrong

17. GL DT DD EV AP IN
    vs ps us gu   Right Wrong

18. GL DT DD EV AP IN
    vs ps us gu   Right Wrong

19. GL DT DD EV AP IN
    vs ps us gu   Right Wrong

20. GL DT DD EV AP IN
    vs ps us gu   Right Wrong

21. GL DT DD EV AP IN
    vs ps us gu   Right Wrong

22. GL DT DD EV AP IN
    vs ps us gu   Right Wrong

23. GL DT DD EV AP IN
    vs ps us gu   Right Wrong

24. GL DT DD EV AP IN
    vs ps us gu   Right Wrong

25. GL DT DD EV AP IN
    vs ps us gu   Right Wrong

26. GL DT DD EV AP IN
    vs ps us gu   Right Wrong

27. GL DT DD EV AP IN
    vs ps us gu   Right Wrong

28. GL DT DD EV AP IN
    vs ps us gu   Right Wrong

29. GL DT DD EV AP IN
    vs ps us gu   Right Wrong

30. GL DT DD EV AP IN
    vs ps us gu   Right Wrong

31. GL DT DD EV AP IN
    vs ps us gu   Right Wrong

32. GL DT DD EV AP IN
    vs ps us gu   Right Wrong

33. GL DT DD EV AP IN
    vs ps us gu   Right Wrong

34. GL DT DD EV AP IN
    vs ps us gu   Right Wrong

35. GL DT DD EV AP IN
    vs ps us gu   Right Wrong

36. GL DT DD EV AP IN
    vs ps us gu   Right Wrong

37. GL DT DD EV AP IN
    vs ps us gu   Right Wrong

38. GL DT DD EV AP IN
    vs   ps   us   gu   Right   Wrong

39. GL DT DD EV AP IN
    vs   ps   us   gu   Right   Wrong

40. GL DT DD EV AP IN
    vs   ps   us   gu   Right   Wrong

41. GL DT DD EV AP IN
    vs   ps   us   gu   Right   Wrong

42. GL DT DD EV AP IN
    vs   ps   us   gu   Right   Wrong

43. GL DT DD EV AP IN
    vs   ps   us   gu   Right   Wrong

44. GL DT DD EV AP IN
    vs   ps   us   gu   Right   Wrong

45. GL DT DD EV AP IN
    vs   ps   us   gu   Right   Wrong

46. GL DT DD EV AP IN
    vs   ps   us   gu   Right   Wrong

47. GL DT DD EV AP IN
    vs   ps   us   gu   Right   Wrong

48. GL DT DD EV AP IN
    vs   ps   us   gu   Right   Wrong

49. GL DT DD EV AP IN
    vs   ps   us   gu   Right   Wrong

50. GL DT DD EV AP IN
    vs   ps   us   gu   Right   Wrong

51. GL DT DD EV AP IN
    vs   ps   us   gu   Right   Wrong

52. GL DT DD EV AP IN
    vs   ps   us   gu   Right   Wrong

53. GL DT DD EV AP IN
    vs   ps   us   gu   Right   Wrong

54. GL DT DD EV AP IN
    vs   ps   us   gu   Right   Wrong

55. GL DT DD EV AP IN
    vs   ps   us   gu   Right   Wrong

56. GL DT DD EV AP IN
    vs   ps   us   gu   Right   Wrong

57. GL DT DD EV AP IN
    vs   ps   us   gu   Right   Wrong

58. GL DT DD EV AP IN
    vs   ps   us   gu   Right   Wrong

59. GL DT DD EV AP IN
    vs   ps   us   gu   Right   Wrong

60. GL DT DD EV AP IN
    vs   ps   us   gu   Right   Wrong

61. GL DT DD EV AP IN
    vs   ps   us   gu   Right   Wrong

62. GL DT DD EV AP IN
    vs   ps   us   gu   Right   Wrong

63. GL DT DD EV AP IN
    vs   ps   us   gu   Right   Wrong

64. GL DT DD EV AP IN
    vs   ps   us   gu   Right   Wrong

65. GL DT DD EV AP IN
    vs   ps   us   gu   Right   Wrong

Key:

GL = global	DT = detail	DD = deduction
EV = evaluation	AP = application	IN = incorporation
vs = very sure	ps = pretty sure	us = unsure
gu = guessed		

READING THE PASSAGE

Basically, the critical reading style appropriate for VR passages means looking for the gist of each paragraph and the function of each part of the text. Don't judge the passages. You'll need to overcome the hurdle of reading material that doesn't interest you or expresses opinions contrary to your own. Don't try to memorize details. The majority of the VR questions will focus on the author's purpose and the structure of arguments, and supporting details can be reviewed if needed.

To get an idea of what we mean, what is the gist and what is the function of the first sentence in the two following paragraphs?

> A well-educated electorate is essential to the survival of a democratic society. Since the only way to maintain a high standard of education throughout all levels of society is through an effectively maintained system of public education, our democratic society must devote significant resources to its public education system in order to assure its continued viability.

> A well-educated electorate is essential to the survival of a democratic society. In aristocracies and monarchies, decisions affecting the well-being of society are made by an elite group, while the great mass of people, having no influence on the outcome, can afford to ignore politics. In democracies, however, the ultimate governing authority rests with the people as a whole, who must be able to make informed decisions.

In the first paragraph, the first sentence is a building block—a supporting fact—for the author's conclusion that funds must be devoted to education. But in paragraph 2 the same sentence *is* the author's principal contention, developed and supported by the succeeding sentences: A counterexample and a comparison. Now let's look at some tools that help you to identify the structure and gist.

Keywords

Keywords are words and phrases that identify purpose or structure. You probably respond to Keywords unconsciously already. Critical Reading involves *consciously* noting and interpreting them. This will save time and improve your comprehension. The common Keyword categories follow, in their order of importance. For each category, think of other words and phrases that convey the same type of information.

Keywords	Purpose	Examples
Conclusion	Identify opinions—whether the author's or some other person's—and the author's tone—positive or negative, strong or mild, emotional or objective. These include all judgmental or emotional words	therefore, wrong, must, conclude, perhaps, unhappy
Evidence	Identify support for an opinion—anything indicating an example, authority, definition, history, or analogy	because, illustrates, several reasons, due to
Contrast	Indicate that a shift or change has occurred or is about to take place—whether in opinion or fact. In VR passages, Opinions are often presented as contrasts to other stated views	but, rather than, distinction, opponents say, not, ironically, alternatively
Emphasis	Identify comparative importance or relevance. These include all superlatives (or comparatives when only two things are compared)	most of all, especially, only, best/worst
Sequence	Identify a necessary order at work—by chronology, importance, or some other criterion	first, then, at one time finally, before/after, and, moreover, this, such, not only . . . but also, similarly, too

When you spot a Keyword, be sure you see what ideas are joined or contrasted. Remember that the words here are just examples—you'll know a Keyword by the type of information it conveys. And the Keyword categories aren't mutually exclusive; Contrast, Emphasis, and Sequence clues add details about Conclusions and Evidence.

Paraphrases

Each paragraph will explore a new aspect of the author's purpose, and one paragraph often provides strong clues about what to expect in the next. Paraphrase each important idea as you read, briefly, and in your own words. Paraphrasing is putting the text into your own words, which assures that you aren't "glazing" and clarifies the major ideas in your mind. Consider this paragraph—how would you paraphrase its ideas?

The challenge of building democracy-sustaining institutions is most acute in the countries of Eastern Europe now working their way out of "real socialism," but it is also a central issue for some noncommunist nations in Asia that have spent decades under various forms of authoritarian and dictatorial rule. True, these authoritarian and dictatorial governments have not achieved the degree of penetration of society attained in good part by the communist regimes of Eastern Europe. Neither have they had the propensity to destroy all elements of civil society or to reconstitute only those that served as instruments of the state and its ruling party. Nevertheless, they have been no more hospitable to the growth of many of the institutions and institutional complexes that are associated with democratic political systems and market economies. They too confront a long agenda of institution building before they may be counted as fully formed and functioning democratic societies.

Paraphrase:

_____

_____

Your paraphrase doesn't have to be more than: "for democs, different tasks face Europe and Asia."

What Keywords helped you? *Challenge* and *propensity to destroy* are Conclusion Keywords, and both *most* and *central* indicate Emphasis. *But*, *not... neither*, and *nevertheless* mark Contrasts. Any one of these words alone might not get your attention, but together they make the purpose of the paragraph clear.

Topic, Scope, and Purpose

The author of every passage has a purpose that you can usually identify in the first few paragraphs. By the time you've finished the first third-to-half of the passage, you should have noted three elements:

Topic—the author's broad subject matter

Scope—the specific aspect of the topic that interests the author

Purpose—why the author has written the passage

All VR passages can be described using one of the following five purposes (be alert for paraphrases of them in the questions):

- Describe   Analyze   Compare   Advocate   Rebut

Two Helpful Statistics:

- In two-thirds of all VR passages, the main idea is stated (or restated) in the last paragraph.
- In half of all VR passages, the first sentence of a paragraph gives you its gist.

Structure

The structure of a passage is its organizational framework: Where is a particular idea introduced? How does it relate to the previous idea? The author chooses a *structure* that imposes order on content to produce a persuasive, logical argument—to accomplish the author's *purpose*. So you'll find that certain structural patterns tend to emerge, based on which purpose the author wishes to pursue.

Verbal Reasoning essays often follow the classic essay formula for college essays:

> introduction — thesis — counter-thesis — synthesis — conclusion.

However, unlike most other standardized admissions tests, MCAT VR uses extracts from published sources for its passages—it doesn't have them written for the test. What's more, in selecting their excerpts, the test makers may lop off introductory and concluding material, or even excerpt material from only one section of the "classic" formula—this is one reason VR passages can be unlike the reading you're accustomed to. If you do see a classic pattern, use it—it will make your reading easier—but *don't assume* there'll be a classic pattern.

HANDLING THE QUESTIONS

As we've seen, the AAMC question categories are:

Comprehension:	Global—main idea, author's purpose
	Details—answers stated expressly in the passage
	Deduction—inferences and assumptions
Evaluation:	Identify the function of a statement or the structure of the passage
Application:	Apply ideas in the passage to new information
Incorporation:	Apply new information to arguments made in the passage

Since the AAMC likes to vary its language, you'll have to watch for paraphrases, like assumption questions worded "what idea is implicit in the author's argument" or "in making this argument, the author relied on which of the following statements."

The skills you need to develop to answer VR questions include:

- Paraphrasing the question to disclose its standard type
- Researching the passage using your map
- Predicting an answer
- Eliminating "pathological" wrong answer choices (see below).

Argument Dissection

Critical reading takes you a long way toward scoring points on VR, but most of the questions you'll face will require more than finding, paraphrasing, or categorizing the appropriate text; they'll require that you understand arguments. In Verbal Reasoning, an *argument* simply means:

> a *conclusion*, or *what* someone wants or believes, plus
> its supporting *evidence*, the reasons *why*.

Don't be misled by the word *conclusion*—it can appear in the beginning, middle, or end of a passage or paragraph. The skills you'll need when a question calls for Argument Dissection include:

- Dissecting the structure of a written argument,
- Identifying the implied part of an argument, and
- Restating each argument in consistent, simplified form.

 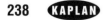

Answer VR questions based on the passage—not based on outside knowledge. Remember, since outside information is not relevant in the VR section, evaluating an argument will never require that you decide whether the evidence is true—just that you evaluate the structure of the argument itself.

VR Arguments have four possible parts:

Part	Function
Opinion	stated conclusion
Facts	stated evidence
Inference	implied conclusion
Assumption	implied evidence

Note that you'll find only two or three of them in any single argument—there won't be both an Inference and an Assumption in one argument. As used here, *Facts* and *Opinions* mean the parts of the argument that you find in the text, rather than the implied Inferences or Assumptions.

The strongest arguments are those with conclusions that *must* be true if the evidence is true. For example:

Evidence: All Central High School volleyball players are over six feet tall, and Sally plays volleyball for Central High.

Conclusion: Therefore, Sally is over six feet tall.

Don't allow your own biases to mislead you when answering VR questions. An argument can be strong even if you reject its conclusion, or weak even if you believe its conclusion is true.

The Stated Parts of Arguments

Isolate Fact from Opinion Using Keywords

Read the following paragraph, then decide whether it's Fact or Opinion or a combination of the two:

> It is misleading to say that advances in communication have made it possible for people to be "better informed" about world events than was possible in the past. There's a limit to how much total information any person can absorb; so the only result of better communications is that, whereas people used to know a great deal about the few places that concerned them directly, now they know very little about a great many places.

Fact _____   Opinion _____   Combination _____

The paragraph generally expresses an Opinion about the nature of information and people's capacity to absorb it, but the statement "There's a limit to how much information any person can absorb" is given as Fact supporting the Opinion that follows it, which is introduced by the conclusion Keyword *so*—therefore, it's a combination. No Keyword labels the evidence, but the context distinguishes it—it's offered as an answer to the question "why should I believe the author's Opinion?" *Misleading* is a strong, judgmental word indicating the author's Opinion in the first sentence. In the second sentence, *only* is Emphasis, and *whereas...used to* and *now* indicate Contrast, which is reiterated in the details: "A great deal about a few places" contrasts with "very little about a great many places."

Note that, as in this case, you may find more than one conclusion in a single paragraph, not just the Opinion that represents the paragraph's principal argument. And often you'll have to dissect one of these subarguments rather than the principal argument.

Now try identifying the argument parts in this paragraph:

> While this may be the most commonly held belief, more enlightened scholars argue that these figures are actually Shinto religious images. They point out that Shinto artists often borrowed Buddhist iconography, so an image that resembles a lion cannot unequivocally be interpreted as a Buddhist piece. Furthermore, Shinto art characteristically displays a peculiar appreciation for the wood (reflecting the belief that a deity may reside in any natural object) and the artist who sculpted these statues carefully followed the natural direction of the wood grain in sculpting curls of the mane and the curves of the forelegs.

The first sentence is the conclusion. It's what the author wants you to believe. If the sentence said simply "other scholars argue" this could be evidence, citing one branch of scholarship on the topic. But the author describes these scholars as "more enlightened"—and that's the author's Opinion. The Keyword *While* prepares you for the second half of the sentence contrasting with the opening clause. Keywords *argue* and *actually* further identify the Opinion. You can see that it isn't necessary to recognize every Keyword, since they often reinforce each other throughout passages.

The second sentence is evidence identified by the Keywords *they point out that*—this is some of the supporting detail provided by the experts. Notice the subconclusion, introduced by *so*—the Opinion of this group of scholars, supported by the Fact that Shinto artists borrowed from Buddhist iconography.

The third sentence is more evidence—as the word *Furthermore* indicates.

Isolate Fact from Opinion Using Context

Often we rely on the context to distinguish Fact from Opinion: Depending on the context, the same sentence can be either a conclusion or evidence. To prove this, identify the function of the italicized statement in the following argument:

> *My apartment is a mess.* My refrigerator is empty. I haven't done laundry in a month. I'm the world's worst housekeeper.

In this case, *My apartment is a mess* is evidence (together with a lot of laundry and an empty refrigerator) for the conclusion that this writer is a bad housekeeper. The first three sentences answer the question, "Why should I believe that this person a bad housekeeper?" You realize this, as you read, as soon as you get through the second sentence: The empty refrigerator doesn't relate to the messy apartment. Since these two statements don't fall into any relationship with each other, they must each relate to something else in the paragraph—each of them does relate to the concept of "housekeeper."

Now identify the function of the same statement in the next argument

> *My apartment is a mess.* The living room needs to be vacuumed. The sink is full of dishes. Dust completely fills the space under my bed.

What has changed? Here, the author concludes that the apartment is a mess based on the evidence in the next three sentences: The apartment has a dirty living room floor, a sink full of dishes, and dust—all aspects of the mess. Remember, the Opinion should answer the question, "what is the author's point?" The Facts should answer the question, "why should we believe the Opinion is true?"

Restate the Argument

When you know what Facts support which Opinion, restate the argument in your own, simplified words:

> The author believes the Conclusion *because* of the Evidence.

This will give you a consistent form to work with, whatever the questions ask. With practice, this step will be automatic and instantaneous by Test Day—saving, not using, time.

Sorting the Opinion from the Facts, restate the argument made in the following paragraph:

> The "Robber Baron" industrialists of the late 19th and early 20th centuries are often portrayed as having no interest in the well-being of society as a whole in their ruthless pursuit of power and personal fortunes. Quite apart from the incidental benefits they provided to society through industrial development, this view ignores the philanthropic endeavors with which most of the Robber Barons were associated. Admittedly a good deal of their philanthropy took the form of bequests; still, these industrialists are responsible for many of our best museums and symphony halls, and the foundations they established continue to rank among the most important sources of charity to this day.

Argument: _____

You probably used different words, but the basic idea is: These industrialists were better than most people think *because* they developed industry *and* because they were very philanthropic.

Note that this argument is never affirmatively stated in the passage: It's expressed as a rebuttal of a common opinion, with the author's opinion apparent in the words *this view ignores*. *Quite apart from* indicates that the first part of the sentence—about the industrial benefits the Robber Barons provided—is in contrast to the more significant evidence—that their philanthropy is sufficient to redeem their reputations. *Admittedly* is another evidence Keyword; you *admit* facts that weaken or refute your conclusion. Although we discuss many of the Keywords present in our passages, remember that you shouldn't worry about catching every Keyword—they reinforce each other, and you only need to note enough to grasp the flow of the argument.

The Unstated Parts of Arguments

Assumptions

The process of deciphering what the author implies is deduction, and Deduction questions are the most common type on MCAT Verbal Reasoning. A VR Assumption is unstated evidence—specifically, a connection between the Facts and Opinion that the author must believe is true in order to reach the stated conclusion. Read the following argument, and write the assumption on the line below.

> Sally plays volleyball for Central High School; therefore, Sally must be more than six feet tall (assuming that ...)

Assumption: _____

The Keyword *therefore* tells us that "Sally is more than six feet tall" is the conclusion, so "Sally plays volleyball..." is supporting evidence. But what's missing?

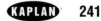

All those who play volleyball for Central High are more than six feet tall.

This Assumption directly links the evidence to the conclusion, and it must be true if the conclusion follows from the stated evidence. Note that either Fact could have been left unstated in this argument: If you are told: "All volleyball players for Central High are more than six feet tall, therefore Sally must be more than six feet tall" then the author must be assuming that Sally plays volleyball for Central High.

Now identify the Opinion, Facts, and Assumption in a more subtle argument:

The company president should allow the office to remain open late, instead of closing at 6:00; much more work would get done. . . .

Opinion: _____

Facts: _____

Assumption: _____

To find an argument's Assumption, focus on the differences between the terms of the evidence and conclusion. In this case, observe that the office doesn't do the work, employees do—so the missing connection between the number of hours the office is open and the amount of work that gets done is the behavior of the employees.

Opinion: The office should be kept open late.

Facts: More work would get done.

Assumption: Employees will be productive for more hours if the office is open longer.

This Assumption directly links the evidence to the conclusion, and must be true if the conclusion follows from the stated evidence. The author's Opinion in this case is identified by the word *should*; the Facts contain no Keywords. Often either the Facts or the Opinion will have Keywords, but not both. So finding the Opinion may be, in part, by process of elimination from the Facts (or vice versa).

Inferences

A VR Inference is an implied part of an argument that must be true if the Facts are true. Consider the following:

Sally plays volleyball for Central High School. All of Central High's volleyball players are more than six feet tall (therefore we can infer ...)

We can infer that Sally is over six feet tall. We are given Facts that necessarily add up to this conclusion. Note the difference between an Inference and an Assumption: The former is a conclusion supported by the given Facts, the latter is an unstated Fact necessary to support the stated Opinion. They aren't interchangeable parts. If you were told:

Sally plays volleyball for Central High School *and* (rather than "therefore") Sally is more than six feet tall

you wouldn't be able to infer that "all volleyball players for Central High School are over six feet tall" as you did in the exercise on Assumptions; it's only a possibility. The information given doesn't support that statement as a conclusion.

 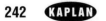

important aspects of the theme of self-discovery. Also, no mention is made of contrasts between Baldwin's early and later work. **C** is FUD—the relationship between racial identity and self-awareness is mentioned at the end of the first paragraph as one aspect of self-discovery. Although the author discusses the relationship between self-discovery and group experience in the third paragraph, she does not "argue" that self-discovery *cannot* take place outside a supportive community, as **D** suggests.

22. D
Although the answer choices seem to contain the bulk of the information in this question, refresh your grasp of the author's major opinions.

LEAST/EXCEPT/NOT questions can be confusing because of their focus on the negative—and the test makers depend on the Opposite answer choice misleading many test takers. Take advantage of the built-in annotation by confirming the answer choice you've selected against the capitalized word.

Choice **D** is the one factor which does *not* contribute to Baldwin's portrayal of self-discovery outlined in the passage. A "commitment to personal independence" contradicts paragraph 2, which says that self-discovery involves an understanding relationship with others; a commitment to *personal* independence would seem to exclude such relationships. Since paragraph 2 stresses compassionate understanding of others as a necessary part of self-discovery, both **A** and **B** are true, and therefore neither is the correct answer. **C** is Opposite, because the author suggests in paragraph 1 that suffering or personal hardship is integral to self-discovery.

23. D
A "definition-in-context" is either an Inference or an Assumption; either you are given all the Facts necessary to infer the definition; or the definition is an assumed Fact, without which the conclusion is invalid.

The question asks about the phrase's meaning in the context of the passage. Be careful not to rely on your understanding of a phrase from its common usage (that will be one of the wrong answer choices, and Outside the Scope of the passage).

Look for the answer to this inference question in paragraph 2, where the phrase "spiritual communion" is found. In the sentence that follows, the author talks about compassionate understanding of others, so the phrase "spiritual communion" seems to suggest a metaphor for gaining insight into others through the spirit of compassion, as opposed to seeking understanding alone. Choice **D**, "sympathetic insight into others," best expresses this thought, and is the correct answer. **A** can be rejected

because the author never discusses religious worship as a theme in Baldwin's fiction—this is an Outside the Scope trap for those who look for the common usage meanings of the words. **B** is incorrect because racial issues are neither specifically mentioned nor implied in the context of the discussion of "spiritual communion with others" in paragraph 2. An ability to endure suffering, choice **C**, is mentioned as an aspect of self-discovery in paragraph 1, where the author never mentions relationships with others.

24. D
Here you are *not* asked what *poignant* means, but what Facts make the word appropriate in this context. But the same method applies; use the immediate context surrounding the phrase or word in question to answer this question about why the author finds the novel "poignant."

Beale Street is mentioned in paragraph 3, as providing an example of a family that finds "selfhood and strength through community." Choice **D** captures this; the novel's poignancy lies in its portrayal of a united community overcoming hardship. **A** is Opposite; it contradicts the novel's theme of the individual uniting with the community to fight adversity successfully. **B** is Outside the Scope; the author never addresses any hardships specific to the Black community. **C** is FUD or Outside the Scope—the author mentions the family's support for the individual, but we don't know whether the Rivers family is traditionally structured or not, so *Beale Street* could hardly illustrate a need for *traditional* family structure.

25. B
An "idea" that is "implicit" is an AAMC paraphrase for an Assumption. A VR Assumption is unstated evidence—specifically, a connection between the Facts and Opinion that the author *must* believe is true in order to reach the stated conclusion. Focus on the differences between the terms of the evidence and the terms of the conclusion. The Assumption directly links the evidence to the conclusion, and *must* be true if the conclusion follows from the stated evidence.

Since the last paragraph focuses on the interrelationship between the individual and the community, **B** provides the most reasonable assumption. **A**, on the other hand, raises the issue of social reform in the black community, a topic which the author never discusses—it's Outside the Scope. **C** is a Distortion and Outside the Scope of the paragraph; it overemphasizes suffering, which the author describes as only one aspect of the process of self-discovery, and it sharply digresses from the third paragraph's discussion of community experience. **D** is Opposite; it contradicts the main idea the passage in suggesting that self-discovery and community identity are incompatible; the very end of the third paragraph says that this isn't the case.

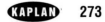

Passage VI (Questions 26–30)

Topic and Scope: Mayan writing, specifically, deciphering Maya signs.

Paragraph structure: Paragraph 1 introduces the two types of Maya writing—logographic and syllabic—which allowed their texts to communicate detail. In paragraph 2 the author expands on the flexibility of Maya writing, showing how certain words can be expressed either logographically or syllabically. In paragraph 3 the focus shifts to the current state of research into Maya signs. Paragraph 4 expresses confidence that the pace of phonetic decipherment will increase in the future despite one factor that may make the process more difficult.

Handling this passage: This fairly dense passage is highly structured. The key to handling a passage like this is keeping track of the progression of the paragraphs.

Think like a test maker: When you see terms defined, like "ahaw" and "pakal" in paragraph 2, you can be sure that at least one question will focus on those terms. Note the author's optimism about the future of phonetic decipherment of Maya texts, which is hinted at in paragraph 3 and expanded upon in paragraph 4. Note in paragraph 4 that the author mentions a potential obstacle to the phonetic decipherment—at least one question will test your understanding of what the obstacle is and how it can be overcome.

26.   C

Deduction questions ask you to identify implied elements of the argument—what must be true based on the information in the passage. Never answer on a hunch—research the relevant text from the passage before moving to the answer choices.

The author discusses what enabled the Maya to write "detailed texts" in paragraph 1. If you've kept track of the paragraph structure, locating it should be easy. In this case, the author notes that "the combination of consonant-vowel symbols and logographs" is what allowed the Maya to include a lot of detail in their texts, so **C** is correct. Choice **A** is FUD; it mentions logographs but doesn't consider syllabic signs. Choice **B** is a Distortion of the idea that one concept can be expressed by more than two signs in Mayan; the author never suggests that one sign can express two subjects. Also, **B** refers to text from the wrong paragraph—paragraph 2, which details how logographic and syllabic signs contributed to flexibility. Choice **D** is a correct statement but FUD, since the author's discussion of allographs in paragraph 4 is irrelevant to the writing of detailed texts described in paragraph 1.

27.   C

Another Deduction question. Mine the question stem for clues as to where the relevant details are discussed in the passage. When inferences or new information constitute the answer choices, always review the relevant opinions before reading the choices. Wrong answer choices will include statements by the wrong party in the passage, or statements on a different point, which it would be easy to confuse with the correct choice without this "regrounding" on the relevant point.

In this case, the word *ratio* in the question stem should point you to paragraph 3's reference to "relative proportions." In that paragraph, the author notes that the relative proportions of logographic to syllabic signs can't be stated because many Maya signs remain undeciphered. The author implies that more work must be done before this ratio becomes clear. Choice **C** states this clearly. **A** is Outside the Scope; the author never discusses the failure of any theory to attract attention. **B** is a Distortion; the author's predictions for increasing decipherment would seem to imply that the ratio may eventually be established. Similarly, **D** is wrong because the author never suggests solving the problem using a "small but representative number of signs."

28.   D

The key to this type of Evaluation question is to consider the context in which the relevant detail appears in the passage: what are the Facts, and what are the Opinions? Remember that, the easier the question stem seems, the trickier the wrong answer choices might be.

The words *ahaw* and *pakal* are discussed in paragraph 2, which describes the flexibility of Mayan by showing that both words can be written in logographic and syllabic form, so **D** is correct. **A** is a Distortion; the author's example shows the different forms in which a word can be expressed, not how many different meanings it can have. **B** is another Distortion; logographic signs are not more flexible than syllabic ones—both types, taken together, create flexibility. **C** refers to the difficulty of understanding Maya texts, discussed in paragraph 4, making it FUD.

29.   D

For this Evaluation question, remember to consider the context in which the detail at issue was presented. Watch out for choices that distort the author's ideas.

The line reference points us to paragraph 3, which focuses on the current state of the decipherment of Mayan. The recent date of discovery of the syllabic structure is there to suggest that the half-completed grid should not be considered unimpressive, as **D** states. **A** is Outside the Scope: There is nothing to suggest that standards today are more exacting. **B** misinterprets the comparison between the time it would take to fill in the syllabic grid and phonetic decipherment. Paragraphs 3 and 4 say that filling in the grid depends on the rate of phonetic decipherment; so both processes are time-consuming. You can eliminate **C** because you can't infer that the half-completed grid will take another 30 years to fill.

30.   C

The correct answer to a Deduction question will not stray far from the passage. Remember to eliminate choices that distort the passage text or seem to come from left field.

The author discusses allographs in paragraph 4; the process of identifying them may complicate, and slow down, the process of phonetic decipherment, although the author believes that the rate of phonetic decipherment will increase in the future, Choice **C**. **A** is Distortion of the last line of the passage. The fact that variant spellings exist for the same word hardly means that scribes couldn't agree on correct spellings. Choice **B** is incorrect because variation in spelling doesn't imply irregular grammar. **D** is a Distortion; the author suggests in the last paragraph not that each allograph is unique, but that each allograph consists of two signs which have the same value.

Passage VII (Questions 31–35)

Topic and Scope: The author's argument against private property

Paragraph structure: The first paragraph argues against any form of compulsion in determining what work men do. The second argues that Socialism is tainted with "authority," which the author considers related to "compulsion." The third paragraph describes the current connection between Individualism (which the author sees as a goal) and private property (which frees those who have it from any compulsion to work). The fourth paragraph expresses the author's view that Individualism for all mankind (rather than for a few persons) will benefit from eliminating private property.

Handling this passage: This is a very formal, even old-fashioned writing style—a type that can be encountered in MCAT VR. Be sure that you read some material from older works, as well as contemporary writers, in your preparations. The politics of this passage are also unpopular today, but don't let your differences of opinion (or your agreement) with the author distract you from the quality and nature of the arguments made.

Think like a test maker: When two people, ideas, or theories are presented within the first paragraph of a passage, ask yourself why the author chose to include more than one viewpoint—to support one over the other, to claim that both are valid or invalid, or to reconcile them?

Establish the purpose of the comparison ad the rest of the passage should fall into place. In this case, the author establishes his ironic tone immediately by contrasting the idea of the enslavement of the few with the idea of enslavement of everyone. Once you get past the dated prose, this is actually a very simply structured argument. This author's Keywords include his verbs (*regretted* and *must be left quite free* and *tainted*), adjectives (*childish* and *arbitrary* and *fine*), adverbs (*I hardly think* and *seriously*) and all other word choices. With so many Opinions offered, you know you'll find questions asking the differences between them.

31.   A

There are five common purposes in VR passages. Whenever a question calls for the author's purpose or intent, you can predict an answer based on synonyms of *to describe, to analyze, to compare, to advocate, or to rebut*. And remember that a vertical scan of the verbs can reduce the number of choices you have to read in full.

Pick up on the author's tone as well as his stated Opinions. Two of the four answer choices here offer positive purposes (*advocating* and *proposing*) while two offer negative purposes (*rejecting* and *refuting*). The number of choices you have to read in full can be cut in half immediately.

The words *primarily concerned* require that you identify the author's overall purpose in the cited paragraphs. This may not be explicitly stated. In the first two paragraphs, the author rejects "slavery," "compulsion," and "authority," which support choice **A**. Choice **B** is a Distortion: "Voluntary organizations" are not advocated by the author. He says only that whatever "associations" men have should be voluntary. **C** is Opposite; the author ironically refers to a scenario in which each citizen "did manual labor for eight hours" as something not even the authoritarian Socialists would want. While the author refers to our handling of "criminals" as done "in a very arbitrary manner," he does not discuss any reform proposals here—**D** is Outside the Scope.

32.   D

This Evaluation question asks you to identify the function of a detail in the passage—you should identify where it is located in the passage and consider its context. Whenever you see a list in a passage, you can expect a question about its function—the longer the list, the greater the likelihood that question will appear.

These five poets are mentioned in the third paragraph as examples of "men who have had private means of their own," who have the "immense advantage" of being "relieved from poverty." In fact, the entire paragraph is there to demonstrate the current benefits of private property—so **A** is Opposite and **B** is Outside the Scope. **C**

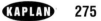

is also Outside the Scope, because the author never discusses what he means by this phrase.

33.   B

This Application question asks that you identify a parallel between the answer choice and some detail or argument in the passage. Review the relevant passage text and identify the broad outlines, the essential elements, of the text. Predict the general structure of the "analogous" choice. Roman Numeral questions require you to consider each of three options before you can determine the correct answer choice. Consider the numeral that appears in the greatest number of answer choices first.

Where does the author refer to "enslaving the entire community"? Does he mean this literally, or is some specialized meaning assigned? As we've noted, this author is speaking simply and literally. Item II matches his intent: The example of Cambodia describes a situation in which everyone is forced to work. In South Africa most people (the Black majority) were enslavedæfiguratively, if not literallyæbut some people (the White minority) were not. Sweden is an example in which no one is enslaved: People simply pay taxes, which is Outside the Scope of the author's argument.

34.   B

Note that in eliminating answer **D** for question 31, you started the review process for this question—another example of one question helping with another.

A and **C** are rather extravagant statements that the author does not make in the passage. (And your answer should be based only on information in the passage. If you feel, personally, that someone who questions our system of criminal justice is likely to be an anarchist, you have to keep that opinion from influencing your choice.) Choice **D** is a Distortion; the author's point is that only when we've determined someone is a criminal do we feel justified in using "compulsion" in connection with him—not that the criminal is in any way suited for such labor.

35.   D

Hypotheticals in question stems may be lengthy and confusing; *before reading their details*, identify what the question asks—will you be looking for an analogy in the passage, or assessing the effect of the new information on the author's argument?

You don't have to know anything about Baudelaire; just refer back to where he is mentioned. The argument there, simply stated, is that some people have been able to "realize" themselves fully because they were freed from any compulsion to work by their private property. Baudelaire is one of five poets mentioned in support of that conclusion. What is the effect if the statement proves untrue with respect to him? There are only four supporting examples instead of five—the logic of the argument is unaffected.

Choices **A** and **B** attribute opinions to the author that he never expresses. The author does make the claim **C** says he does, but the information in the question stem does not strengthen it—It's FUD. This information does not affect the validity of the author's other supporting examples, so validity of the main argument is not affected.

 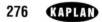

CHAPTER NINE

Writing Sample

Medical schools want an assessment of your reasoning and written communication skills—your essays should be critical, not emotional. You'll be writing two essays for the MCAT, each in response to a stimulus, and each within a half-hour.

Your essays will be graded on a scale of 1 to 6, with Level 6 being the highest. Graders will be looking for an overall sense of your essay, not assigning separate scores for specific elements like grammar or substance. They realize you're writing under time pressure and expect you to make a certain number of mistakes. Two readers read each essay and score them independently. If the two graders differ by more than a point, a third grader is a final judge. Those scores are added together, and the combined score is converted into an alphabetical rating ranging from J to T. Statistically speaking, there will be few Level 6 essays. An essay of 4 or 5 would place you at the upper range of those taking the exam.

WHAT SKILLS ARE REWARDED IN THE WRITING SAMPLE?

The AAMC lists the following as the skills tested in the Writing Sample:

- Developing a central idea
- Synthesizing ideas
- Presenting ideas cohesively and logically
- Writing clearly

The first of these involves having a central idea that unifies your essay, the second and third mean tying all your ideas together logically. The fourth skill is the only one addressing your writing skills directly, and it's limited to clarity. This is not principally a test of your writing—the AAMC wants a chance to see your reasoning skills.

The skill that the AAMC didn't mention is speed. The skills listed here would be relevant if you were writing an essay over the course of several weeks. On the MCAT, you have to do all this, but in 30 minutes. This can't be done using the same procedures you have learned to use for essay writing in the past.

DO YOU NEED TO PREPARE FOR THE WRITING SAMPLE?

Like the Verbal Reasoning section, this section tends to be underestimated by MCAT test takers. Most think they can just apply their everyday writing skills to the MCAT—a dangerous assumption. Every section of the MCAT is a test of analytical reasoning—even the Writing Sample.

The Writing Sample is not like other writing experiences. It's a first draft, but one that will be graded. It must not only be complete and well organized, but also easy for a grader to see that it is complete and well organized (the grader may spend as little as 45 seconds on an essay).

The MCAT essay is one of the very first things the admissions person sees and thus will be part of your "first impression." The MCAT essay is read *often* and by *most* medical schools. If a medical school is on the fence about you, the quality of the essay may help make the decision.

Practicing the MCAT Writing Sample also strengthens your Verbal Reasoning skills. (Naturally! In the Writing Sample you're putting together an argument. In VR, you're taking arguments apart. The one skill will inevitably complement the other.) Don't try to cut corners. Learn the Kaplan Method. Practice writing at least one essay a week. Make the Method yours. If the essay is great, it can only help you. If it's weak, it can only hurt.

ESTABLISH AND ADHERE TO A PRACTICE SCHEDULE

Rough Calendar

Just as we said about Verbal Reasoning, the Writing Sample is a section for which you have to internalize methods and strategies, and for which no last minute cramming will be effective. If you intend to maximize your score, you must establish and adhere to a practice schedule. Start practicing essay writing, using the Kaplan Method, right away, and do it methodically throughout your study period.

Writing Essays

There is no substitute for practicing writing essays based on as many of the AAMC released items as possible (you'll find them in your *MCAT Announcement*). Time yourself to internalize the pacing necessary to complete the tasks. Never start to write until you have a complete Prewrite, and then adhere to your Prewrite. Always reserve two minutes to look over the essay and make needed corrections.

Scoring Your Essays

Basically, there are four criteria for scoring the Writing Sample essay: did you address the tasks, is the essay organized, have you presented and developed any ideas, and have you used language effectively. The score you can earn based on accomplishing these goals is indicated in this chart:

 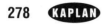

	1	2	3	4	5	6
Tasks	none	some	some	all	all	all
Organization	none	none	some	some	strong	strong
Ideas/Depth	none	none	clear	clear	depth	depth
Language	confusing	confusing	coherent	coherent	coherent	flowing

A 1 essay misses all the tasks, is disorganized, has no coherent ideas, and makes many spelling or grammatical errors. A 2 essay is only superior in that it at least addresses one of the tasks, however superficially. A 3 essay does contain ideas, uses language in a coherent manner, and is organized, although there are digressions.

A 4 essay addresses all three tasks, but is otherwise a 3 essay. A 5 essay addresses all three tasks in some depth and with strong organization.

The skill that distinguishes a 5 essay from a 6 essay is superior use of language; but this doesn't mean that you have to use any particular style or vocabulary. If you know your strengths, and avoid your weaknesses, all you have to do is vary your sentence length and structure and have your ideas flow naturally from one to another in order to score a 6.

Outside Reading

Your practice reading for Verbal Reasoning will also help develop your reasoning and writing skills for the Writing Sample. After reading pieces expressing opinions or contrasting two or more views, flex your capacities to analyze and state divergent views, by asking yourself:

How would this have sounded ten years ago? 50 years ago?

What groups or people would disagree, and why?

What philosophy underlies this?

What would be an even more extreme restatement of this?

The Kaplan Method for the Writing Sample

Step 1: Read and Annotate

Step 2: Prewrite First Task

Step 3: Prewrite Second Task

Step 4: Prewrite Third Task

Step 5: Clarify Main Idea and Plan

Step 6: Write

Step 7: Proofread

The Kaplan Method emphasizes the Prewrite—these few minutes make the biggest difference in both completeness and organization of your finished essay. If you Prewrite using the Kaplan Method, and adhere to your Prewrite when you write, your essay will be solidly organized. Between now and Test Day, you can't drastically change your overall writing skills—and you probably don't need to. If your Prewrite is good, all you need to do in the writing and proofreading steps is draw on your strengths and avoid your weaknesses. Get to know what those are as you practice.

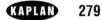

Maximizing Your Score

To streamline your view of how to maximize your score, let's look at what the AAMC tells you about how the essays are scored, and reduce the requirements for each higher level to those elements not shared with the prior level. Doing this, we get:

To score Level 4, the AAMC requires that you:

- Address all three tasks
- Show logical thought and organization, but nothing very complex
- Demonstrate strong skills in word use

To score Level 5, all you have to add to a Score of 4 is:

- Interpret the statement in some depth
- Present a fairly organized essay

To score Level 6, all you have to add to a Score of 5 is:

- Use sophisticated language and strong organization

Since Kaplan's Prewrite will ensure solid organization, the difference between a 4 and a 5 comes down to "depth," and the difference between a 5 and a 6 is the way your use of language ties your ideas together. Let's explore what this means, using the following "skeleton" of the AAMC Writing Sample statement (without the details of a specific "statement"):

> Write a unified essay in which you perform the following tasks:
> Explain what you think the above statement means. Describe a specific
> situation in which … . Discuss what you think determines when… .

To earn a score of 4, your essay has to fulfill each task—in other words, you have to follow the instructions. Before Test Day, you should become familiar with these "general" instructions. Many scores are lower than they could be simply because one or more of these standard directions are violated. Words in the instructions that students often overlook or misread in Writing Sample essays are:

The operative verbs for each task: *Explain, describe,* and *discuss*

The words *you think* in Task I (you're asked for a personal view; you're not being tested on your knowledge of the subject)

The word *specific* in Task II (no generalities or vague examples; be sure that your example in Task II is more specific than the others, since specificity is expressly called for there)

And, finally, don't overlook *unified* in the first line of the directions.

In the context of the general Writing Sample directions, following instructions (and earning at least a score of 4) means:

On Task I: *Explain* what the statement means *to you.*

On Task II: *Describe* a *specific* counter-example.

On Task III: *Discuss* the *criteria* for tasks I and II.

With that in mind, what do you think could be added to each of the tasks in order to add the "depth" required for a score a 5 on each essay? We suggest:

Describe an *example*.

Explain the *relevance* of your counter-example.

Resolve the apparent contradiction between your Task I and Task II discussions.

Kaplan has found this approach useful in its many years of experience with hundreds of sample Writing Sample statements. Notice that we've simply switched the verbs in Tasks I and II—each task can be developed by drawing on the kind of detail requested in the other. Concrete examples clarify your thinking about each task. And although they only mention them in Task II, the AAMC graders love specific examples. No matter how familiar your example is, don't rely on the grader's knowing why and how it is relevant; state your reasoning.

Now, according to the AAMC, a score of 6 means language is used in a sophisticated way—each idea flows naturally and sensibly from what came before it. With that in mind, what would you add to each of the tasks in order to score a 6? We suggest:

Use an effective *hook* to bring the reader in.

Regular *transitions* provide the glue that holds your ideas together.

End with a *bang* to make your essay memorable.

To make your ideas flow naturally, give your essay a clear introduction, a distinct middle section, and a strong conclusion. You make it easier for the grader to follow your logic if you insert appropriate Keywords of the types you learned to recognize in Verbal Reasoning: Evidence, Conclusion, Contrast, Emphasis, and Sequence of ideas (but avoid the most overused and obvious ones, such as *for example*, which appear in most essays). A "hook" means avoiding an essay that opens (as thousands of other essays will) "The statement means...." A "bang" means a closing that ties the three paragraphs together. Good choices for either can be a clear, succinct statement of your "thesis" in the essay or a vivid example that's right on point.

Why the Writing Sample Is So Difficult

Kaplan has found that it's common for students to have trouble quickly coming up with content, in enough detail and sufficiently interconnected, to produce a unified, balanced essay. This happens, in large part, because of the nature of the WS "statement"—it is extreme, therefore inherently weak and difficult to work with.

Consider this sample statement, for example:

An artist should not be influenced by the public's judgment of his or her own work.

This can be understood as: An artist *absolutely should not at any time* be influenced by *any of* the public's judgment of *any of* his or her own work. That statement can be pretty hard to defend, so ideas explaining or supporting it may not occur to you. What can you do?

The "First Task" shouldn't necessarily be Task I—in fact, depending on the nature of the stimulus, you will probably find it easier to start with Task II, which is inherently less extreme—and for some, it's simply easier to argue than to agree! In applying the Kaplan Method, make the "First Task" the one that's easier for you, then use those ideas to help you develop the other two tasks. To the extent that ideas *do* occur to you immediately in response to a statement on Test Day, use them—the graders appreciate originality and a fresh approach. But when you've mastered the

Kaplan Prewrite process described in this workshop you can go into the MCAT confident that you can develop an essay regardless of the topic.

Reliable Criteria

Instead of approaching the MCAT statements in isolation, start with some criteria in mind that will help to shape your thinking. In its many years of MCAT experience, Kaplan has found four reliable criteria for use in Writing Sample essays:

> Survival/Safety
>
> Time
>
> Size/Demographics
>
> Education

These are not the only possible "general" criteria you might use; but they have been carefully chosen. They tend to be fairly neutral. You could base your essays on your moral convictions (assuming you have any related to the statement), but drawing on strong, emotional convictions is not the best way to produce a balanced, reasoned essay in a short time.

What do these criteria mean, and how can they assist you in the free association process needed to draw together sufficient detail to build your essay? We can explain this best with an example. Consider whether it is "good" to burn leaves, based on each of the Kaplan criteria. Note your thoughts briefly.

Based on Survival/Safety: _____

Based on Time: _____

Based on Size/Demographics: _____

Based on Education: _____

Some possible thoughts are:

For survival/safety: Individually, the danger of burning yourself, locally, the danger of the fire spreading, environmentally, the danger to the ozone layer—can you think of more?

For time: Compare the attitude in the nineteenth century, or even the 1950s, with our attitude today, or compare different times of day, or different times of year—others?

For size/demographics: Consider the danger of a single fire to the danger if everyone burns their leaves, or the danger if I burn my leaves compared to the burning going on in the Amazon jungle—what else?

For education: Understanding the risks determines when, how, and where leaf burning is appropriate; what about education on the effects of burning toxic leaves (like poison ivy)—can you think of other knowledge or understanding that is relevant?

Using Kaplan's standard criteria as one of your starting points improves your Prewrite in two ways; it stimulates more ideas, and unifies those ideas because they all shared a common focus.

 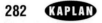

APPLYING THE KAPLAN METHOD

Now let's apply the Kaplan Method to the following practice Writing Sample statement:

Consider this statement:

> An artist should not be influenced by the public's judgment of his or her own work.

> Write a unified essay in which you perform the following tasks: Explain what you think the above statement means. Describe a specific situation in which an artist should be influenced by the public's judgment. Discuss what you think determines when an artist should and should not be influenced by public judgments of his or her work.

Step 1: Read and Annotate

(One-half minute or less)

First, be sure you see *precisely* how Task II should vary from Task I: Should your counter-example demonstrate that every artist should be influenced by public judgments; that artists should *sometimes* be influenced by public judgments; or that *some* artists should be influenced by some public judgments?

Next, aside from being sure you follow the general instructions as we discussed earlier, highlight and define words that are abstract, subjective, or ambiguous—or for which you'll use a limited or expanded meaning. You don't need The-One-Right-Definition for any word in the statement. You just want to make clear to the graders how you are using the words in your essay.

What if you don't know "artists" well enough to identify examples? You don't need to! Draw on what you do know about. Use the term artist—and any other terms in the statement—as broadly as you need to. Use TV writers or sports figures as "artists"—or you can even make one up: Your good friend Bob Santiago is a great artist; he can also be a politician, or actor, or anything you're comfortable writing about. The WS essays do not test specific knowledge. You aren't graded based on the nature of your examples, as long as they are responsive to the tasks. But remember, if you decide to treat a term unusually, be sure to define it!

Consider what *public* means—is it unambiguous? Will you use it in a particular sense? Even if you are using a common definition, fix it in concrete terms—you shouldn't switch between *public* as in "public park" meaning "communal" (but there may be rules and restrictions on its use) and *public* as in "public information" meaning "freely and unrestrictedly available to all."

Will you investigate what *judgment* is and how the *public's judgment* is to be known?

Exploring one or two terms in the statement will contribute significantly to the graders' perception of "depth" in your answer.

Step 2: Prewrite the First Task

(One minute or less)

In college composition classes, many of you learned to "brainstorm"—perhaps using a "clustering" approach to organizing your ideas. These are excellent strategies if you have the luxury of days or weeks to write your essay. They lead to unbalanced, disorganized essays if you have to write in a half hour. Kaplan's Prewriting system is designed to produce balanced and integrated essays in the 30 minutes allotted on the MCAT.

We'll start with Task II, but the same process will apply if you start with Task I.

> **An artist should not be influenced by the public's judgment of his or her own work.**

To meet the requirements we established to maximize your score for Task II, we will need to:

II. 1. *Describe* a *specific* counter-example.

2. Explain the *relevance* of your counter-example.

3. Use regular *transitions* to keep the essay unified.

Decide which of the "reliable" criteria leads most naturally to an example of when an artist *should* be influenced by the public. It can help to imagine that the statement presented is made by the most irritating person in your life; how would you respond? Even if you really agreed, you might be tempted to argue.

In this case, we chose to use the criterion of "survival" and the example of "an unknown artist who has to support himself." That's the kind of note you should be making for yourself as you Prewrite. You can't write out the sentences yet: you won't have time to write them twice, and you shouldn't be composing sentences until you have decided what the whole essay is about—not just one paragraph.

The answer we've chosen is that, based on the need to survive, the artist has to be influenced by public opinions when the artist needs to establish an audience. Other possible answers might be "when the work is for a public building" (based on "demographics") or "when the artist works in a totalitarian state" (based on "survival" in a different sense)—you may have come up with something entirely different. Draw on your own knowledge—this isn't a test of your knowledge of any specific art or artists.

Next, working with our proposed response, comb your memory (or your imagination) for an example of an artist working to establish himself. We'll use:

example: imaginary blues singer supports himself performing old standards

relevance: income from works the audience already knows

Filling in the details mentally (the task calls for a specific example) we'll call the singer Noah Peyton, who can't perform his own, highly original compositions until he wins a recording contract. Jot down any notes you need to ensure that you use the details you've developed.

Note that you can't complete the third "Score Maximizing" item until you turn to Task I and determine how much, and on what basis, your Task I and Task II paragraphs will differ. Don't be afraid to skip around in your Prewrite, filling in the pieces as they occur to you. If you have a good Task III example or an idea for a conclusion, note it now rather than risk forgetting it.

Even using the same criterion, your example is probably very different. For now, let's continue with ours.

 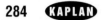

Step 3: Prewrite the Second Task

(One minute or less)

Since we started with Task II, the "Second Task" is Task I. As we found in our "Score Maximizing Checklist" we will need sufficient detail in our Prewrite to:

I. 1. *Explain* what the statement means *to you.*
   2. Describe an *example* to provide depth.
   3. Use an effective *hook* to bring the reader in.

The concrete example chosen for Task II and the "reliable" criterion selected from Kaplan's list give you additional information to approach this task. With them in mind, how will you interpret the statement? We chose:

art for its own sake, artistic integrity requires that the artist ignore others' opinions

And what example can you think of or invent to add depth? We chose:

Frederick Shoen, who is wealthy, can devote himself to pure artistic expression

Again, we've invented an answer. Fill in the details in your mind, making notes only as needed to ensure that you don't lose your ideas. You may not be ready to decide what your opening "hook" will be until you've developed ideas for the entire essay. Come back to this if you don't have any ideas now.

Now that you have most of your Prewrite for Task I, return to Task II and fill in appropriate transitions. The ideas we've developed so far suggest that we favor artistic integrity, but we're aware of times in an artist's life when survival requires compromise; our transition should reflect these ideas. How might you connect the second paragraph to the first? We'll use:

At times, though

You might prefer "But this isn't always possible ..." or an opening that uses your counter-example immediately, like "Noah Peyton, on the other hand ..." or something completely different that you've seen in a Verbal Reasoning passage. Whatever you choose, be sure it conveys your meaning effectively—establishing quickly how your second paragraph relates to the first and how it will differ from it.

If you find that you need additional detail for a balanced essay, add depth to your essay by answering the *hard* questions:

What is the *history* of either side?

What *assumptions* underlie either side?

What is the *relevance* of an example?

What are the *differences* between persons or groups holding these opinions?

Step 4: Prewrite the Third Task

(One minute or less)

To maximize your score on this task, our goals are:

    III. 1. *Discuss* the *criteria* for Tasks I and II.

        2. *Resolve* the apparent contradiction.

        3. End with a *bang* to make your essay memorable.

Notice that by satisfying items 1 and 2 you will automatically tie this paragraph closely to the first two paragraphs.

    criteria: need for money, career goals and status

    resolution: first survive, then art

This is our shorthand for the idea that, you can't serve your artistic integrity by starving to death early in your career, so eating has to come first (but of course the artist does continue to practice his art to whatever extent possible in the meantime). Now you have everything you need to select your opening and closing. We've chosen to start with:

    I. 3. Purists want artistic independence

and to close with:

    III. 3. The artist must balance goals

Step 5: Clarify Main Idea and Plan

(One minute or less)

Now take a moment for two decisions before you start to write:

1. Do you intend to agree with the statement or counterstatement, to take a position in-between, or to remain neutral? This will determine the tone of your opening and the types of additional transition words you'll use. Don't agonize over this decision, though. This doesn't have to be your opinion for life—just an argument you can present logically, based on the details you've developed.

2. Where will you discuss any terms in the statement that need explanation or clarification? This will usually be done in the first paragraph (which may therefore be a little longer than the other paragraphs), but be sure you discuss a term where it's most relevant and best contributes to the overall flow of your ideas.

Finally, based on those decisions:

- Cross out ideas that you now consider superfluous to your essay,
- Number the points you want to make, in the order you think will be most effective, and
- Start to select Keywords you'll use for clear connections and transitions.

Make transitions smooth and clear with the same Keywords that you use to identify the author's argument in Verbal Reasoning. But the graders will appreciate it if you avoid the most obvious and overused ones, such as *for example* and *thus*.

Step 6: Write

(23 minutes)

Use one paragraph for each task, so your essay will be easy for readers to follow. Don't get emotional—graders don't care what you think, they care how you think.

Write in your mind before you write on paper. The three paragraphs of your essay will in fact be organized around the three "topic sentences" which you should finish *in your mind* before you start to write:

- The statement means...
- One example of when the statement is wrong is....
- The factors that determine whether the statement is applicable are...

You should generally avoid actually writing these sentences in your essay (the graders see thousands of essays that do recite these words), but completing these sentences *in your mind* ensures that you are addressing each of the tasks.

Given the time constraints imposed by the Writing Sample, it's vital to the clarity of your writing that you use the ideas and organization you established in the Prewrite. Resist any urge to introduce new ideas or to digress from the central focus or organization of each paragraph.

A few common weaknesses to keep in mind:

- Avoid using "I"
- Avoid cliches, slang, and redundancy
- Vary sentence length and structure to give your essay a rhythm

Write neatly. Graders will be prejudiced against your Writing Sample if it's hard to decipher. If this is a problem for you, print your essay.

Step 7: Proofread

(2 minutes)

Always leave yourself 2 minutes to review and edit your work—the time spent in this way will definitely pay off. Very few of us can avoid the occasional confusing sentence or omitted word when writing under tight time limits. Quickly review your essay for blatant errors or significant omissions. You don't have time to revise substantially. Learn the types of mistakes you tend to make and look for them. Some of the most common mistakes in WS essays are:

- Sentence fragments
- Subject-verb agreement errors
- Misplaced modifiers
- Pronoun agreement and consistency errors
- Misused words—especially homonyms like *their* for *there* or *they're*
- Spelling errors

Don't hesitate to make corrections on your essay—these are timed first drafts, not term papers. But use a minimum of marking for clarity: A single line through deletions, and an asterisk marking text to be inserted and the place to insert it.

YOU BE THE GRADER

Let's look at an essay based on our Prewrite. When you've read it, decide what holistic grade you would give it.

Art has been at the center of many debates throughout history. What is art? What does it mean to be an artist? What function should art and the artist play in society? One interesting debate about art focuses on the very source of art—an artist's inspiration. Some argue that art should be created for an audience and that the artist should cater to the audience's tastes and desires. Others counter that art should be created for art's sake, that an artist should be inspired from within, and create works that express the artist's creative vision and serve his artistic integrity. If artists cater to public opinion, they argue, they are creating not works of art, but instead pieces of entertainment. Art, they believe, serves not merely to entertain, but also to inspire, inflame, soothe, and express. Arguing against public influence on art, purists point to painters like Willem van Lees, whose early works pointed to a great artistic talent and a potential for artistic innovation and upheaval in the world of fine painting. Van Lees, though, fell victim to public influence and the wealth that accompanied public approval, and faded into relative obscurity as a portrait painter. In contrast, Van Lees' associate, Frederic Shoen, independently wealthy and inspired by Van Lees' early works, created works that were not popular with contemporary audiences but today hang in prominent museums as examples of true artistic innovation and inspiration.

At times, though, an artist should seek public approval for his own work, even if such approval comes at the (temporary) expense of his artistic integrity. One such circumstance is the case in which the artist needs to gain widespread exposure so that a larger audience could appreciate his work. Noah Peyton was a struggling blues singer in the early 1980s. After giving up his job as a school custodian, Noah set out to obtain a recording contract so that he could release a selection of songs he had written over the years. No recording companies wanted to invest in a relatively unknown singer and his songs at the time. Noah began to perform at small parties, clubs, and festivals. At these venues, the audience wanted to hear old blues standards rather than Noah's original compositions. While gaining a small following of fans over a few years, Noah's own works were overshadowed by popular requests. When Noah did finally get a recording contract a few years later, the recording company only allowed him to record two original compositions. After several successful releases of cover songs, Noah was finally able to release a collection of his own songs.

So, there are times in which an artist should ignore public opinion and times in which an artist should embrace public input. What factors come into play? The motive of the artist in creating his works is an important consideration. If an artist wishes merely to entertain, then public opinion should be a factor in a piece's creation. If an artist wishes to serve his artistic integrity, he should listen only to his "inner artist." Long-term and short-terms goals should be considered. Frederic Shoen, financially comfortable in the short-term, was in a good position to ignore public demand and focus on art for art's sake. Noah Peyton, on the other hand, had to subordinate his own artistic desires to the public will in the short term in order to gain the popularity that would allow his original compositions to reach a larger audience. In the end, an artist must decide what he wants to accomplish with his work.

Score: _____

ANALYSIS OF THE SAMPLE ESSAY

This is an essay by a confident writer, and reads pretty well for a first draft. You might have been tempted to give it a 6—but it doesn't merit it. In some respects, there are so many levels of meaning and so much density that it was hard for the writer to keep track of the point being made. Let's review it closely (but remember that this is not how the graders will view it, and any one of these problems individually would not cost the author points).

> Art has been at the center of many debates throughout history.

This is a very general opening that could be eliminated without loss of meaning or clarity. Since time is so short, it's best to avoid empty sentences; but don't worry if you've opened this way—in itself it won't cost you points.

Our first comment is on the appearance of the essay as a whole—at a glance, the grader would assume that the three tasks are not equally treated, since the paragraphs decrease in length as the essay continues. Without making it an obsession, try to keep your three paragraphs fairly equal in size.

> What is art? What does it mean to be an artist? What function should art and the artist play in society?

Avoid rhetorical questions unless you feel you do have a strong point to make and can make it without leaving any loose ends. Rhetorical questions can be effective, but you have to be sure that you develop the answers fully—if you don't, this format will call attention to the omission, and make it seem worse than it really is. In this case, the last question (about the function of the artist in society) runs the additional risk of confusing the topic of the essay, which is supposed to be about the effect of society on the artist, rather than vice versa.

> One interesting debate about art focuses on the very source of art—an artist's inspiration. Some argue that art should be created for an audience and that the artist should cater to the audience's tastes and desires. Others counter that art should be created for art's sake, that an artist should be inspired from within, and create works that express the artist's creative vision and serve his artistic integrity.

The author gives both sides of the issue here; that can be a good strategy, but it also requires careful follow-up. In this case, the author doesn't clearly tie the second paragraph back to this dichotomy; so it's not clear that a consistent argument is being made in the two different paragraphs.

> If artists cater to public opinion, they argue, they are creating not works of art, but instead pieces of entertainment.

It's clear that the author considers "entertainment" inferior to art, but the terms are never clearly defined or developed. You may have to define terms that you introduce to the discussion, as well as terms used in the statement.

> Art, they believe, serves not merely to entertain, but also to inspire, inflame, soothe, and express.

Here, again, the author throws out too many ideas, and fails to make them consistent. If art is to "inflame" and "inspire," isn't the public judgment relevant? The author has to resolve this issue if these ideas are kept in the essay. Leave out terms you don't have the time (or the knowledge) to explain and clarify.

> Arguing against public influence on art,

Here's a subtle example of why you should define the terms of the statement, and use them consistently. If the word *influence* were not one of the terms in this statement, this might be a fair paraphrase. But the statement says "public judgment" should not "influence" the artist—and the reference to "public influence" here collapses the two terms, raising the risk that the author (and the grader) will get confused.

> purists point to painters like Willem van Lees, whose early works pointed to a great artistic talent and a potential for artistic innovation and upheaval in the world of fine painting. Van Lees, though, fell victim to public influence and the wealth that accompanied public approval, and faded into relative obscurity as a portrait painter.

This is a classic Writing Sample miscalculation. The author is presenting an example for Task I in the negative; essentially, the example is someone who *did* let the public judgment influence his art, and was hurt by it. What about an example of why *not* being influenced by public judgment is *beneficial* to the artist? Particularly when the statement is expressed in the negative, avoid increasing the chance of confusion by a negative example. (This example might have been reworked for the third paragraph, with proper discussion of its relevance.) Note, too, that that the author didn't stick to the Prewrite—this idea came to mind while writing and wasn't well-developed.

> In contrast, Van Lees' associate, Frederic Shoen, independently wealthy and inspired by Van Lees' early works, created works that were not popular with contemporary audiences but today hang in prominent museums as examples of true artistic innovation and inspiration.

This second example in the first paragraph is the one that should have been used exclusively; the one who produces great art by ignoring the public's opinion. But it is given comparatively little space and development because of the focus on the negative example.

> At times, though, an artist should seek public approval for his own work, even if such approval comes at the (temporary) expense of his artistic integrity. One such circumstance is the case in which the artist needs to gain widespread exposure so that a larger audience could appreciate his work.

This is a good, clear statement of the contrary view. The only quibble with this sentence (and by itself it wouldn't cost points) is that "At times..." is sufficient without the "(temporary)" inserted later.

> One such circumstance is the case in which the artist needs to gain widespread exposure so that a larger audience could appreciate his work.

This statement is not clear; fortunately, the detailed development of the example that follows makes the meaning clear, but this sentence adds nothing except possible confusion.

> Noah Peyton was a struggling blues singer in the early 1980s. After giving up his job as a school custodian, Noah set out to obtain a recording

 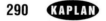

contract so that he could release a selection of songs he had written over the years. No recording companies wanted to invest in a relatively unknown singer and his songs at the time. Noah began to perform at small parties, clubs, and festivals. At these venues, the audience wanted to hear old blues standards rather than Noah's original compositions. While gaining a small following of fans over a few years, Noah's own works were overshadowed by popular requests. When Noah did finally get a recording contract a few years later, the recording company only allowed him to record two original compositions. After several successful releases of cover songs, Noah was finally able to release a collection of his own songs.

This is a great example, with good detail. But where's the explanation of its relevance to the overall point being made? To make the point clear, a sentence or two should tie this paragraph back to the language used in introducing the two viewpoints in the first paragraph. Since the essay generally includes sufficient depth, this single omission won't mean the essay can't earn a 5.

So, there are times in which an artist should ignore public opinion and times in which an artist should embrace public input.

This sentence is clear, but very general. This can be effectively used, but you have to be sure you follow up on this sentence fully and quickly.

What factors come into play?

Even if the rhetorical questions are well-used in the first paragraph, don't overdo it. Too much rhetoric breaks the "flow" of your ideas; wherever you interject rhetoric, you have to follow through or it calls too much attention to itself and makes the essay look *less* well written than it is.

The motive of the artist in creating his works is an important consideration. If an artist wishes merely to entertain, then public opinion should be a factor in a piece's creation. If an artist wishes to serve his artistic integrity, he should listen only to his "inner artist."

The author introduces the idea of the "motives" of the artist here for the first time. "Entertainment" was mentioned in the first paragraph without development, and with a negative tone. Now it's presented as one of two apparently acceptable goals. Defining terms and having a clear statement of your thesis before you write can avoid this kind of confusion.

Long-term and short-terms goals should be considered.

The addition of a second criterion is excellent, and this one has been developed in the discussion of Peyton.

Frederic Shoen, financially comfortable in the short-term, was in a good position to ignore public demand and focus on art for art's sake.

This ties the paragraph back to the point made about Shoen earlier—an excellent strategy.

Noah Peyton, on the other hand, had to subordinate his own artistic desires to the public will in the short term in order to gain the popularity that would allow his original compositions to reach a larger audience.

The tie-back to Peyton is also well done. One, very subtle consideration: You've discussed a painter and a musician. Are you sure that a reader might not conclude that different art forms require a different result? A few words making it clear that this is not the case might be in order.

> In the end, an artist must decide what he wants to accomplish with his work.

A short statement of conclusion like this can be very effective if you have fully developed the ideas leading up to it.

PRACTICE AND SELF-EVALUATION

There is simply no substitute for writing essays under test-like conditions. Be hard on yourself. Don't allow yourself any extra time to complete an essay, and don't look at essay topics in advance of doing your practice essay. Since the actual MCAT will require you to write two essays back-to-back, you may want to do your practice essays in one-hour sessions. On the other hand, single-topic practice tests may be more useful if you spend time reviewing and scoring each essay immediately after writing it. As part of your self-evaluation, you should determine which method is most useful to you.

Between now and Test Day, practice writing essays based on as many of the AAMC-released items as possible. For each one, give yourself 30 minutes to write the essay. After each practice essay you write, score yourself based on the guidelines provided here. Then analyze how well you followed the Kaplan Method in constructing your essay, and how you might improve on the next. Do you have any tendency to rush your prewrite, or do you find that you haven't left two minutes to proofread? Practice to get your pacing internalized and reliable.

GET A SECOND OPINION

Ask someone else to read and critique your practice essays. If you know someone else who's taking the MCAT, you might agree to assist each other in this way. If your reader doesn't know the MCAT essay section, you may want to show them the student essays and evaluations in the AAMC Student Handbook first. In either case, knowing whether another person can follow your reasoning is the single most important learning aid you can have for the Writing Sample.

WRITING SAMPLE PRACTICE ESSAY

Writing Time—30 Minutes

DIRECTIONS: The first part of this section presents a sample Writing Sample statement. Write an essay in response to the prompt, timing your response and applying the Kaplan Method. Use wide-ruled sheets to write your essay.

Following the prompt is Kaplan's Writing Sample Scoring Guide, an in-depth look at the criteria the MCAT graders will use. Working with the sample statement you have just written about, the Scoring Guide will show you what distinguishes a 6 essay from a 5 essay, a 5 from a 4, and so on.

Please do not look at the Benchmark essays in the Scoring Guide before writing your own essay—that would defeat the purpose. When you *do* look at the Benchmark essays, try to form your own opinion of each essay's merits and flaws before looking at the critique. Doing this will help you develop your own critical skills, a crucial step to becoming a good writer.

Consider the following statement:

Citizens of a democracy must follow the law, whether or not they agree with it.

Write a unified essay in which you perform the following task: Explain what you think the above statement means. Describe a specific situation in which citizens who oppose a law should not follow that law. Discuss what you think determines when citizens who disagree with a law are justified in not following it.

STOP ⬤

WRITING SAMPLE SCORING GUIDE

We've already discussed scoring in simplified terms. This Scoring Guide is a more comprehensive breakdown and discussion of the writing sample score.

A score of **6** indicates that the essay:

- Fully addresses all three tasks
- Presents a thorough discussion of the topic
- Shows depth, synthesis, and complexity of thought
- Has clearly focused and coherent organization
- Has superior vocabulary control
- Has superior sentence structure and variety

As indicated, the first three of these characteristics relate to *content*. You must address all three tasks. The information and examples must be specific to the topic and relevant to the intent of the essay, in a way that's clear to the grader.

The fourth characteristic is *organization*—the arrangement of the content for a coherent sequence of ideas. Each paragraph should deal with a single subject. Transitions between ideas should be logical. The grader should sense the presence of an introduction and a conclusion and should know what's happening at all times in the essay. Digressions should be avoided.

The fifth characteristic concerns *vocabulary*, and clarity and conciseness are the keys. You want to select the best words to get the message across. Incorrect and ambiguous words cause confusion and cloud the message. Inflated and pompous diction is considered a weakness.

The final characteristic relates to *sentence structure*. All statements should be complete in meaning and structure. Fragments should generally be avoided, and sentences (especially the beginnings of sentences) should vary in length and in structure.

A score of **5** indicates that the essay:

- Substantially addresses all three tasks
- Presents some depth, synthesis, and complexity of thought
- Has coherent organization
- Has substantial vocabulary control
- Contains effective sentence structure

A 5 essay is a very good essay but lacks the style of a 6 essay. Technically, it is free of major errors. It does not contain glaring or annoying problems that distract the grader.

A score of **4** indicates that the essay:

- Moderately addresses all three tasks
- Presents a moderate discussion of the topic
- Shows clarity but lacks depth of thought and synthesis
- Is coherent but has digressive organization
- Has overall vocabulary control
- Has controlled sentence structure

A 4 essay is a good-to-fair essay but tends to be pedestrian and dull. Although it addresses all three tasks, it does not go further. The grader might sense that the writer is struggling for ideas and words. A weak organization or some digressions might derail the grader. It is basically free of errors, but its vocabulary and sentence structure lack polish.

A score of **3** indicates that the essay:

- May neglect or distort one or more tasks
- Presents a minimal discussion of the topic
- Shows some clarity of thought but is simplistic
- Has weak organization
- Has minimal sentence control

A 3 essay does not contain all the information required. This essay may allude to, but not really address, one or more of the tasks. It might distort one or more of the tasks. Weak organization, vocabulary or sentence structure may indicate that the writer does not have control of the topic.

A score of **2** indicates that the essay:

- Seriously neglects or distorts one or more tasks
- Presents little, if any, discussion of the topic
- Lacks clarity of thought
- Has confused organization
- Lacks language facility
- Has confused syntax and recurrent mechanical errors

A 2 essay demonstrates a serious deficiency of writing skills. Ideas are either nonexistent or confusing. The weak structure thwarts the grader, who must struggle to make sense of the essay. The essay may contain sentence fragments or excessive spelling or punctuation errors that impede the grader. The student is clearly not a competent writer.

A score of **1** indicates that the essay:

- Does not address the tasks
- Fails to address the topic
- Confuses ideas and thoughts
- Lacks organization
- Confuses vocabulary
- Has seriously flawed syntax and mechanics

An essay that receives a score of 1 is seriously deficient. The writer does not demonstrate an understanding of the topic or competence in writing.

Benchmark Essays

Each of the following Benchmark Essays represents a specific score. The essay is probably not in the top or bottom range for the score, but at the midpoint—the average or typical response for the score.

The sample essays in this Scoring Guide are student essays written by MCAT candidates. Each was read and scored by six trained graders who agreed within one score point. The essays have been typed as written, reproducing all features, including errors. Each Benchmark is followed by a critique that explains its holistic score.

Benchmark 6

The formation of a democracy is, in a sense, "government for the people" in which the citizens of a city, state, or country have some voice in the legislation process. This "voice" is usually constituted in the voting process, where individuals vote for candidates they feel support their views. Thus, when an individual is elected, he or she gained the majority of votes from the public and will hopefully support the views in this population. It is obvious, however, that not all people will be satisfied with the winning candidate. Nevertheless, since they did have a vote in the election and the candidate won by a fair majority of votes, it is the duty of these citizens to accept the winner as their leader. It seems logical, then, that citizens of a democracy follow the law put forth by the leaders of their country (whether they agree or not) due to the manner in which these leaders were elected. if all citizens disobeyed the laws they disagreed with then our country's leaders would surely not have the ability to mandate any laws or attempt to "put them into action," and thus the entire organization and structure of our society would completely disintegrate.

On the other hand, with so many rules there always appear to be exception. There are specific situations in which citizens who oppose a law should <u>not</u> follow that law. A good example is a topic of controversy in current events today—abortion. to many supporters of the "Right to Life" campaign, an abortion is an act which terminates the life of a potential human being. These supporters are fighting in the courts to attempt to make abortion illegal. Unfortunately, the scenario if abortion is made illegal is not a pleasant one. Abortion is a matter of choice and opinion, and who is to say one person's opinion is more correct or lawful or powerful than another's? When a law is passed that actually states how one should treat his or her body, it does not seem necessary to follow a law of that magnitude. It seems logical that a young girl of 16 who accidentally get pregnant while using birth control and is <u>not</u> ready to be the mother of a child should not be <u>forced</u> by the law to bear that child and go through the trauma of attempting to raise it or giving it up for adoption. When a law dictates one's life to such a degree that his/her entire future is at stake, I believe that justification for not following that exists. Now, this broad statement could be applied to many laws, and it could ultimately be argued that many laws are opposable and thus people are justified in not following them. What a catastrophe would result if this type of logic was followed!

It seems that the most realistic conclusion to settle on is that there is no <u>general</u> rule that can be stated as to when a person is justified in breaking the law. However, treating each scenario separately and making one's judgments case dependent would be a fair and honest system to determine such a broad and complex issue.

Critique of the Benchmark 6 Essay

This essay clearly addresses all three tasks. In a thorough presentation, the writer explains the meaning of the statement, describes the contradictory situation of abortion, and discusses the justifications ane ramifications of not following the law. The writer uses strong details and delves deeply into the topic. Althovgh it is not recommended to include controversial topics like abortion in the Writing Sample essay, the author manages to thoughtfully explore this emotional issue.

The writer uses a subtle, controlled style to develop the central idea that laws must be obeyed, but sometimes there are exceptions. However, these exceptions must be dealt with individually and specifically in order to maintain the democracy.

The essay's organization is coherent and focused. The essay devotes a paragraph to each task. Transitional devices are especially effective. Note the use of *Thus*, and *On the other hand*. The essay carries the grader easily from one idea to the next.

Vocabulary is especially appropriate. The first paragraph contains words associated with democracy, such as *voting process, candidates,* and *election*. The writer uses specific terms when describing abortion, such as *"Right to Life"* and *matter of choice* and *opinion*. The overall vocabulary is aptly chosen and powerful, for example, *constituted, mandate, terminates, magnitude, ultimately,* and *catastrophe*. The writer also uses qualifying words to expand on ideas, such as *Nevertheless,* and *However*. Overall, the writer demonstrates good facility of language.

Sentence structure is varied and interesting. Sentences flow smoothly, and occasionally the writer draws the grader into the discussion by asking a rhetorical question or by making an emphatic point.

The essay is largely free of errors, awkward phrasing, and ambiguities that distract the grader.

Note, however, that these three paragraphs vary widely in size. This author has handled the "resolution" of the different sides of the issue in the first two paragraphs, so the final paragraph only has to tie the ideas together. Avoid this structure unless you are very confident about your graders' ability to see that the tasks are each fully treated.

Benchmark 5

The definition involves the notion of "the People's" choice. Every person in a democracy is able to participate in the process of making a decision whether it be to choose a president or amend a law. Therefore, when a law is legislated, it is legislated with the approval of "the people." Of course, the term "the people" is defined a group consisting of millions of citizens all with different views and beliefs. It is impossible for every single person to agree to one point of view. However, in a democracy, the majority rules. If the minority does not agree with a certain law, it still must obey the law because that is how a democracy functions.

In general, this belief holds true for the citizens of a democracy. However there are situations when a citizen should not obey the law. One such situation would involve a law promoting racial discrimination. A law that discriminates against a person because of ethnic origin is a law that should not be upheld. It is a law that degrades, not preserves human dignity. Laws are formed to protect the citizens of a democracy and if one particular law degrades "the people," then they must disobey it. One specific example to strengthen this argument concerns Rosa Parks who refused to leave the white section of her bus. Being forced to stand because she was black would have destroyed her human dignity. She had the right to preserve her dignity. She had the right to disobey the law.

The justification of a broken law is a complex subject analyze. if is difficult because one cannot talk about justice in objective terms. Justice is subjective. To the blacks, Rosa Parks was justified in what she did. To the whites, she was not. Justice is a notion that is contingent on one's own beliefs. For me, as a citizen, to decide if disobedience of a law is justified, I must determine if this law is compatible with my personal beliefs or not. if the law is not compatible with my beliefs, then I must say that disobedience of that law is justified.

Critique of the Benchmark 5 Essay

The key word for a 5 essay is *substantial*. With some careful editing this essay would be improved. The writer clearly demonstrates an ability to discuss the topic and its three tasks. After a substantial affirmation of democracy in the first paragraph, the writer presents the countervailing situation of legalized racial discrimination in the second paragraph. The discussion moves from the general (racial discrimination) to the specific (Rosa Parks's disobeying a segregation law). The conclusion focuses on the implication of a *broken law*.

Organization is coherent. The writer uses transitional phrases (*Therefore, Of course, In general, One example*). Ideas are arranged logically and flow smoothly from one to the next.

Vocabulary is appropriate, if not dazzling. The writer lacks a flair for using words, making the essay rather pedestrian. For example, note the repeated use of *a law*.

Sentence structure is especially effective in the third paragraph where the writer uses a variety of sentences. Effective balance occurs in the sentences beginning with *To the blacks* and *To the whites*.

This essay, however, is not flawless. Redundancies and excessive wordiness characterize many of the sentences. In the last few lines, the writer shifts into the first person, either an awkward attempt to establish a rapport with grader or an unnoticed slip.

Benchmark 4

Citizens of a democracy must follow the law, whether or not they agree with it. The law is created with the citizens in mind, and in most case, it was voted upon by the people. Therefore, since the laws are "confirmed," per se by the citizens, everyone should follow them as well. Laws are for the good of the people. Protecting their rights and freedoms. Protecting them from the most likely result of abolishing law, or chaos.

Even though in most cases, citizens should feel obliged to follow the law, there are some instances when the best thing to do for a citizen who opposes a law, is not to follow it. One example of this could be the draft. According to the law, if you are eligible for the draft and are drafted, you are expected to perform the military services assigned to you. However, if you are opposed to the draft or fighting in a war, it is better not to go, if

 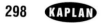

they are prepared to face the consequences. Many men who are drafted and are morally opposes to fight, but go anyway, are the ones who end up shooting themselves in the foot or committing suicide. It is better not to go, if those are your intention, We need men willing to defend our country in the military, not those who are constantly looking for a way out.

This does not mean that in general, when a person is opposed to a law they should not follow it, because then as stated earlier chaos would be the result. Instead, I feel that there are factors that determines when citizens who disagree with a laws are justified in not following it. It depends on the severity of the law, and its underlying purpose. The law which sets the limit for blood alcohol level and intoxication was made to protect citizens from doing damage to themselves, as well as others, and willfully breaking such a law and operating a motor vehicle is asking for trouble.

Critique of the Benchmark 4 Essay

In the Benchmark 4 Essay, the writer *moderately* addresses all three tasks, but not thoroughly or substantially.

The essay begins with a discussion of democracy. This first paragraph, however, is characterized by blanket statement rather than by exploration of ideas. Next, the writer attempts to develop an exceptional case by using the draft as a specific example. The effort is weakened by the writer's lack of logical, concrete argument. Here the writer states that if one opposes the draft and fighting, *it is better not to go* than to fight without motivation. The paragraph ends with a personal sentiment rather than with detailed, convincing argument.

The conclusion unifies the essay by referring again to chaos, thus recalling the idea suggested in the first paragraph. However, with the introduction of a new idea—the law that sets the limit for blood alcohol level and intoxication—the essay becomes digressive.

Except for this digression, the essay is coherently organized. Each paragraph develops an idea that reflects one of the three tasks.

Vocabulary is generally not misused or ambiguous, although pronoun usage in the second paragraph is chaotic. Sentence fragments occur and in one sentence the second person becomes the third. Punctuation is haphazard.

Overall, this essay meets the basic requirements for an acceptable essay.

Benchmark 3

Citizens of a democracy should not believe that there are no reasons for which they should not follow the law. There comes a time when the law no longer applies or protects the people and must be changed. Democracy may be the best government system developed but like all other things human, its not perfect. Unfortunately, to change and modify the law usually requires some drastic demonstration to bring this to the attention of the people as a whose. It is for these reasons that disobedience to the law is sometimes justified.

Early in the history of our country not all men were free. Slavery was legal and very much a part of our society. As a black, you had no rights, not even the right to life. As it has been said there are certain unalienable rights deserved by all men. These specifically are the right to life, liberty, and the persuit of happiness. Slaves too believed that they were deservant of these rights. It took great protest by many whites, constant rebellion by the black slaves, and eventually a civil war to change this law. During this campaign I'm sure I am correct in saying that many disobeyed the law for which did not serve them.

More recently in our history, Martin Luther King spent time in a Birmingham jail in protest to segregation. Here again the black community did not believe the law justly served them and thus could not comply. This is not the only example. Through our history many have been in protest to laws and have suffered the consequences in their efforts to correct the problem. Prior to the American Revolution, many protested the laws and taxes set on them by the English by refusing to comply. It is the right of the people to change their government if it no longer effectively protects it citizens.

Marx said the government that no longer protects its citizen will be overturned and anew government put in its place until it no longer works. This cycle is and endless set of revolutions. Today we find it much easier to change our democracy at a lesser cost to society than revolution. However, strong events demonstrating the uneffectiveness and unjust is usually still the most effective way. It is not until the citizen of a society see the unjust inflicted upon someone that they stir their emotions to act.

On a smaller scale I will pose another question. Is it wrong for someone to steal food for survival when he or she finds no other alternative to come by this. If he does not steal then he may starve, but if he steals he could be punished. And is our law and society just in pursecuting him for trying to survive.

Critique of the Benchmark 3 Essay

This essay exemplifies the demarcation between an acceptable essay and an unacceptable essay because it fails to fulfill the directive. It does not address all three tasks. The first paragraph addresses the topic but does not really define or explain democracy. The first sentence introduces the confusion that continues throughout the essay: "Citizens of a democracy should not believe that there are no reasons for which they should not follow the law."

The paragraphs that follow do not really address the remaining tasks, but instead present a confusing survey of protests. The writer mentions *slaves, the Civil War, Martin Luther King, Jr., the American Revolution, Marx* and his political theory, and finally a starving person who steals food. Discussion of these examples is minimal. As a result, this essay makes no progress in intellectual argument and cannot qualify for any score above a 3.

The essay is showy in its abundance, but shallow and simplistic in its argument. Poorly organized, it moves through history without evident purpose. (Why discuss Martin Luther King before the American Revolution? Why the digressive paragraph on Marx?) One example does not lead naturally to the next to make a point for the grader. Analysis and synthesis are nearly nonexistent.

Vocabulary choice is weak. The essay abounds in unnecessary negatives; the words *no* and *not* seem to dominate the essay. The use of the first person is intrusive and tends to serve as filler. The foggy use of the indefinite form of the pronoun you creates confusion: As a black, you had no right....

Sentences have not been thoughtfully constructed. Many sentence beginnings are verbose; for example, *As it has been said...* and *More recently in our history....* Indeed, whole sentences lack vitality and interest because they are overloaded with excess verbiage. This essay could be reduced by one third without sacrificing any of the writer's ideas.

Benchmark 2

A democratic population is expected to abide by the laws and restrictions and freedom of that society despite its personal conflicts with any particular branch.

A democracy is not always able to voice every individual's opinions and rituals thereby leading to a chaotic environment often chosen by extremists. Such is the case of abortion which has earned an overwhelming public interest over the past couple of decades. Abortion, unless used as a means of birth control, should be left up to the individual who is directly affected by it. There exists a number of reasons which determine why people should not agree with the laws set for abortion. Economy takes the leading role, followed closely by religion. A family's financial situation is the major determinant of abortion. There is no point in bringing a life in this world if proper care is unavailable to the child. Love and nourishment, health of the mind and body are extremely essential for the growth of a baby. This is sometimes very rarely found in single-parent families, not out of the parent's wish but more of the inability due to time inavailability and job demand. Even in families with both parents present, this fast pace expensive world demands both their time and attention in exchange of a little more financial solvency.

Critique of the Benchmark 2 Essay

This essay seriously neglects or distorts the required tasks. The first paragraph feebly attempts to explain the meaning of the essay topic in a single sentence. The structure of this sentence is confused, and the prepositional phrase at the end forces a grader to ask "branch of what?" (end of paragraph 1).

The discussion of the topic centers on abortion. The writer devotes the remainder of the essay to this issue. Despite a promise to review the financial and religious reasons that precipitate some abortions, the writer discusses only financial reasons and ends the essay before completing the second and third tasks.

Organization is especially weak since the essay lacks a conclusion. The writer does not analyze the ramifications of disobeying a law or achieve any synthesis of opposing ideas. In fact, the central ideas are not logically connected.

Diction is elementary and often incorrect. For example, the writer combines an *individual's opinions and rituals* as the object of the verb *voice*. Vocabulary, too, is misused, as in *abide by...freedom*.

Frequently, sentences are convoluted or awkwardly phrased; for example, "love and nourishment, health of the mind and body are extremely essential for the growth of a baby". Unclear or incorrect linkages (e.g., "thereby leading") make it difficult to follow the writer's train of thought.

Overall, this essay represents the writing skills either of an inexperienced writer who failed to plan and ran out of time or of a poorly trained writer who has not mastered the ability to organize prose.

Benchmark 1

Since the beginning of history and man, people have been abiding a set of rule's by the community, or being punished for disobeying someone or some law. Citizens in a democracy must follow the law, wheather its good or bad. Every one must believe a democracy irregardless if its good or bad. Many laws upset people and they leave their country. I believe if you are bothered by laws you should vote at every election and talk to people who live in another country. Many of the law's being made have had flaws. Some teenagers do not follow the law and have to pay a price for it. But, if they pay the price they won't be around to make new and better laws when they become adults. I believe a citizen has the right to decide wheather or not he or she should follow it and be ready to accept total punishment for the actions taken, but feels justified by the actions taken. Its a matter of consciousness and being able to cope with the decision you decided to make.

Critique of the Benchmark 1 Essay

This passage completely misses the mark. The writer fails to address the topic and provides little if any concrete information about the tasks. The first sentence introduces the confusion that continues throughout the passage. The writer's reference to *teenagers [who] do not follow the law* suggests an attempt to establish an opposing example, but fails to develop it.

Organization is weak. The one-paragraph structure indicates poor organization, which is confirmed by the internal confusion. For example, there is no unity of ideas as the writer moves from *Citizens in a democracy* to *people who live in another country* to *teenagers [who] do not follow the law*. The writer tends to state convictions rather than discuss and argue concepts.

Vocabulary is nonstandard (*irregardless*, and misused *consciousness*).

Syntax and mechanics are seriously flawed. For example, the sentence "Every one must believe a democracy irregardless if its good or bad." contains numerous errors that cloud its meaning. The author confuses *its* or *it's* and there are erratic pronoun shifts throughout the passage. However, these errors in grammar are not the primary causes of the low score.

How Did We Do? Grade Us.

Thank you for choosing a Kaplan book. Your comments and suggestions are very useful to us. Please answer the following questions to assist us in our continued development of high-quality resources to meet your needs.

The title of the Kaplan book I read was: _____

My name is: _____

My address is: _____

_____

My e-mail address is: _____

What overall grade would you give this book?   (A)   (B)   (C)   (D)   (F)

How relevant was the information to your goals?   (A)   (B)   (C)   (D)   (F)

How comprehensive was the information in this book?   (A)   (B)   (C)   (D)   (F)

How accurate was the information in this book?   (A)   (B)   (C)   (D)   (F)

How easy was the book to use?   (A)   (B)   (C)   (D)   (F)

How appealing was the book's design?   (A)   (B)   (C)   (D)   (F)

What were the book's strong points? _____

How could this book be improved? _____

Is there anything that we left out that you wanted to know more about?

Would you recommend this book to others?   ☐ YES   ☐ NO

Other comments: _____

_____

_____

Do we have permission to quote you?   ☐ YES   ☐ NO

Thank you for your help.
Please tear out this page and mail it to:

    Managing Editor
    Kaplan, Inc.
    888 Seventh Avenue
    New York, NY 10106

KAPLAN®

Thanks!

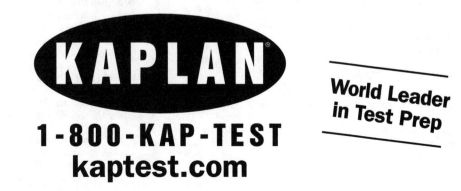

About Kaplan

KAPLAN TEST PREPARATION & ADMISSIONS

With 3,000 classroom locations throughout the U.S. and abroad, Kaplan has served more than three million students in its classes over the past 60-plus years. Kaplan's nationally-recognized programs for roughly 35 standardized tests include entrance exams for secondary school, college and graduate school as well as English language and professional licensing exams. Kaplan also offers private tutoring and one-on-one admissions guidance and is a leader in test prep for computerized exams. Kaplan is the first major player to provide online test prep to students across the globe, as well as admissions courses and other resources at **www.kaptest.com.**

SCORE! LEARNING, INC.

SCORE! Learning, Inc. is a national provider of customized learning programs for students. *SCORE!* Educational Centers help students in K-10 build confidence along with academic skills in a motivating, sports-oriented environment after school and on weekends. *SCORE!* Prep provides in-home, one-on-one tutoring for high school academic subjects and standardized tests. *SCORE!* Educational Centers and *SCORE!* Prep share a highly personalized approach, proven educational techniques, and the goal of cultivating a love of learning in children.

THE KAPLAN COLLEGES

The Kaplan Colleges system (**www.kaplancollege.edu**) is a collection of institutions offering an extensive array of online and traditional educational programs for working professionals who want to advance their careers. Learners will find programs leading to bachelor and associates degrees, certificates and diplomas in fields such as business, IT, paralegal studies, legal nurse consulting, criminal justice and financial planning. The Kaplan Colleges system includes Concord Law School (**www.concordlawschool.com**), the nation's only online law school, offering J.D., Executive J.D. and LL.M. degrees for working professionals, family caregivers, students in rural communities, and others whose circumstances prevent them from attending a fixed facility law school.

QUEST EDUCATION CORPORATION

Kaplan's Quest Education unit (**www.questeducation.com**) is a leading provider of post-secondary education. Quest offers bachelor and associate degrees and diploma programs designed to provide students with the skills necessary to qualify them for entry-level employment. Programs are primarily in the fields of healthcare, business, information technology, fashion and design.

KAPLAN PUBLISHING

Kaplan Publishing, in a joint venture with Simon & Schuster, publishes more than 150 titles on test preparation, admissions, education, career development, and life skills. Kaplan Publishing emerged as a leader in sales of books for statewide assessments with the publication of dozens of new state test titles. Books are offered in traditional paper form, pre-packaged with computer software, and now in e-book form.

KAPLAN INTERNATIONAL

Kaplan International (**www.kaptest.com**) provides students and professionals with intensive English instruction, university preparation, test preparation programs, housing and activities at 12 city and campus centers in the U.S. and Canada. Kaplan also has a strong presence overseas with 41 centers in 18 countries outside of the United States.

KAPLAN COMMUNITY OUTREACH

Kaplan Community Outreach provides educational resources and opportunities to thousands of economically disadvantaged students annually. Kaplan joins forces with numerous nonprofit groups, educational institutions, government agencies, and other grass-roots organizations on a variety of local and national support programs. These programs help students and professionals from a variety of backgrounds achieve their educational and career goals.

KAPLAN PROFESSIONAL

The Kaplan Professional companies (**www.kaplanprofessional.com**) provide licensing and continuing education, training, certification, professional development courses, and compliance tracking for securities, insurance, financial services, legal, IT, and real estate professionals and corporations. Offering an array of educational tools, from on-site training and classroom instruction to nearly 200 online courses and programs, Kaplan Professional serves professionals who must maintain licenses and comply with regulatory mandates despite busy travel schedules and work obligations.

- **Dearborn Financial Services** provides innovative education and compliance solutions to the financial services industry, including registration services, firm element needs analysis and training plan development, securities and insurance prelicensing training, continuing education, and compliance management services, in classes nationwide, online and via books and software.

- **Dearborn Trade Publishing** publishes approximately 250 titles specializing in finance, business management and real estate, plus well-read consumer real estate books to help homebuyers, sellers and real estate investors make informed decisions.

- **Dearborn Real Estate Education** is the leading real estate content provider for real estate schools and associations, offering practical prelicensing and continuing education training materials on appraisal, home inspection, property management, brokerage, ethics, law, sales approaches, and contracts, and an online real estate campus at **RECampus.com.**

- **Perfect Access Speer** is a leader in software education and consulting, bringing both traditional and e-learning solutions to its clients in the legal, financial, and professional services industries.

- **The Schweser Study Program** offers training tools for the Chartered Financial Analyst (CFA®) examination, with a comprehensive product line of study notes, audiotapes, videotapes, flashcards and live seminars that are developed and taught by a top-notch faculty.

- **Kaplan Professional Real Estate Schools** provide real estate licensing and continuing education programs through live classroom instruction, Internet-based learning, and correspondence courses, to help real estate professionals acquire the skills needed to meet state licensing and educational requirements.

- **Self Test Software** is a world leader in exam simulation software and preparation for technical certifications including Microsoft, Oracle, Cisco, Novell, Lotus, CIW and CompTIA, serving businesses and individuals seeking to attain vendor-sponsored certification.

- **Call Center Solutions** provides assessment and training services to the call center industry.

Want more information about our services, products or the nearest Kaplan center?

1 Call our nationwide toll-free numbers:

1-800-KAP-TEST for information on our test prep courses, private tutoring and admissions consulting

1-800-KAP-ITEM for information on our books and software

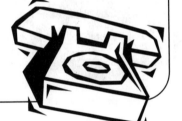

2 Connect with us online:

On the web, go to:
www.kaptest.com

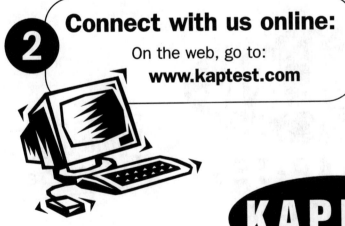

3 Write to:

Kaplan
888 Seventh Avenue
New York, NY 10106

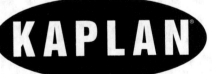

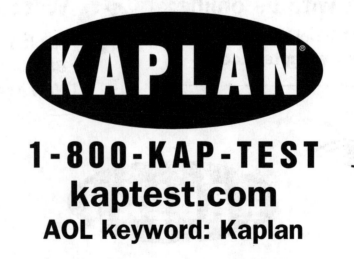